Praise for *Healthy Places, Healthy People, Third Edition*

"The third edition of *Healthy Places, Healthy People* begins with the principle that the health of people begins with the health of their community. This text takes providers out of hospitals and clinics and into the culture of communities—into workplaces, schools, homes, and neighborhoods—where health is both created and compromised. The authors assume that to work with communities, you have to know how communities work, their political and economic realities, their strengths, their frailties, and their capacity for mobilizing citizens for action. This how-to book, grounded in an understanding of culture and all its complexity, provides realistic strategies and practical advice for achieving health equity."

—Bechara Choucair, MD
Senior Vice President Safety Net & Community Health
Trinity Health

"*Healthy Places, Healthy People* is a masterfully written text for nursing students learning about community health nursing. The art of nursing includes understanding the communities where people live their lives. This text exposes the learner to the importance of understanding the patient in the larger context of community through a culturally informed lens. Nursing professionals in all areas of nursing practice would benefit from reading the third edition of *Healthy Places, Healthy People* to fully understand what scope of care means along the entire healthcare continuum."

—Monica Dillon, RN
Community/Public Health Nurse
Loyola University Community Nursing Center

"This book is a well-designed text that identifies community as keeper of culture, dynamic, and defined from the inside, while setting out the different skills and competencies that promote leading change and social justice. It includes concrete examples and materials that can be used in completing a community culture assessment, a theoretical model that can guide a culturally focused community practice of nursing. Integral is a well-defined understanding that culture is not about ethnicity and that the meaning of community entails how space and time is used. The meaning of community is found in lifeways and manners in which people are organized and interact. A must-read for any practitioner interested in true community engagement and change."

—P. Ann Solari-Twadell, PhD, RN, MPA, FAAN
Associate Professor and Director, Global Health Experiences and International Studies
Marcella Niehoff School of Nursing, Loyola University Chicago

"This book weaves together public health nursing practice, culture, and social justice, emboldening nurses to place values into practice. Its thoughtful organization allows for concise yet visionary descriptions of strength-based and community-based theoretical approaches, practice examples, and case studies. This edition brings to life a holistic public health nursing care that will inform undergraduate students' practice for years to come."

–Angela Kueny, PhD, RN
Assistant Professor, Luther College

"The authors of *Healthy Places, Healthy People* are pioneers in the practice of culturally informed healthcare, and this book serves to capture their enormous practitioner experience in a refreshingly new academic framework. As a person who has been using this model for many years, I can say with confidence that this book fills a much-needed gap and will be very useful for practitioners and students around the world."

–R. Balasubramaniam, MD, MPhil, MPA
Founder, Swami Vivekananda Youth Movement, India
Former Frank Rhodes Professor, Cornell University

"The third edition of *Healthy Places, Healthy People* provides the reader with practical strategies to lead change and promote social justice in healthcare. This handbook is applicable to more than just nursing. Individuals in all healthcare settings striving to promote a healthy society can benefit from reading this guide. As a nurse scientist, I have used the culturally informed strategies outlined in this text in recruitment and will continue to reference this guide when engaging in communities."

–Fayron Epps, PhD, RN
National Hartford Center of Gerontological Nursing Excellence
Claire M. Fagin Fellow 2013–2015

"*Healthy Places, Healthy People* provides a groundbreaking, very adaptable framework for community/public nurses at any stage of their career. This edition is even more streamlined and is an excellent resource for classroom instruction, research studies, and practice projects. This handbook has had an enormous influence on my professional practice as a nurse practitioner in the care of individuals and communities."

–Mandy Peacock, DNP, AGPCNP-C

HEALTHY PLACES, HEALTHY PEOPLE
THIRD EDITION

A Handbook for Culturally Informed Community
Nursing Practice

Lisa Elaine Skemp, PhD, RN, FGSA, FAAN
Melanie Creagan Dreher, PhD, RN, FAAN
Susan Primm Lehmann, MSN, RN

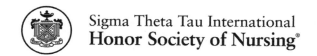

Sigma Theta Tau International
Honor Society of Nursing®

Sigma Theta Tau International
Copyright © 2016 by Sigma Theta Tau International

The Honor Society of Nursing, Sigma Theta Tau International (STTI), is a nonprofit organization founded in 1922 whose mission is to support the learning, knowledge, and professional development of nurses committed to making a difference in health worldwide. Members include practicing nurses, instructors, researchers, policymakers, entrepreneurs, and others. STTI has more than 500 chapters located at more than 700 institutions of higher education throughout Armenia, Australia, Botswana, Brazil, Canada, Colombia, England, Ghana, Hong Kong, Japan, Kenya, Lebanon, Malawi, Mexico, the Netherlands, Pakistan, Portugal, Singapore, South Africa, South Korea, Swaziland, Sweden, Taiwan, Tanzania, Thailand, the United Kingdom, and the United States of America. More information about STTI can be found online at www.nursingsociety.org.

Sigma Theta Tau International
550 West North Street
Indianapolis, IN 46202

To order additional books, buy in bulk, or order for corporate use, contact Nursing Knowledge International at 888.NKI.4YOU (888.654.4968/US and Canada) or +1.317.634.8171 (outside US and Canada).

To request a review copy for course adoption, email solutions@nursingknowledge.org or call 888.NKI.4YOU (888.654.4968/US and Canada) or +1.317.634.8171 (outside US and Canada).

To request author information, or for speaker or other media requests, contact Marketing, Honor Society of Nursing, Sigma Theta Tau International at 888.634.7575 (US and Canada) or +1.317.634.8171 (outside US and Canada).

ISBN: 9781940446660
EPUB: 9781940446677
PDF: 9781940446684
Mobi: 9781940446691

Library of Congress Cataloging-in-Publication Data

Names: Dreher, Melanie Creagan, author. | Skemp, Lisa Elaine, 1955- , author. | Lehmann, Susan Primm, author.
Title: Healthy places, healthy people : a handbook for culturally informed community nursing practice / Lisa Elaine Skemp, Melanie Creagan Dreher, Susan Primm Lehmann.
Description: Third edition. | Indianapolis, IN : Sigma Theta Tau International, [2016] | Melanie Creagan Dreher's name appears first in the previous editions.
Identifiers: LCCN 2016013154 (print) | LCCN 2016015817 (ebook) | ISBN   9781940446660 (print : alk. paper) | ISBN 9781940446677 (epub) | ISBN   9781940446684 (pdf) | ISBN 9781940446691 (mobi) | ISBN 9781940446677 (Epub) | ISBN 9781940446684 (Pdf) | ISBN 9781940446691 (Mobi)
Subjects: | MESH: Community Health Nursing | Culturally Competent Care | Transcultural Nursing--methods
Classification: LCC RT98 (print) | LCC RT98 (ebook) | NLM WY 106 | DDC   610.73/43--dc23
LC record available at https://lccn.loc.gov/2016013154

First Printing, 2016

Publisher: Dustin Sullivan
Acquisitions Editor: Emily Hatch
Editorial Coordinator: Paula Jeffers
Proofreader: Todd Lothery
Interior Design and Page Composition: Rebecca Batchelor

Principal Editor: Carla Hall
Project and Development Editor: Kezia Endsley
Copy Editor: Heather Wilcox
Indexer: Larry D. Sweazy
Cover Design: Rebecca Batchelor

DEDICATION

This book is dedicated to the citizens and students who have shared with us the joy and struggle of building sustainable, healthy communities and promoting social justice and health equity.

ACKNOWLEDGMENTS

We are deeply indebted to the communities in which we work and the people and groups that have opened their doors and hearts to students from the University of Massachusetts, University of Iowa, Rush University, and Loyola University–Chicago, who have embraced a new way to nurse and enthusiastically set about working with community members in creating healthier places for people to have healthier lives.

The treatise of this text is easily traced to Columbia University Teachers College and the Department of Anthropology, where Professors Lambros Comitas and Conrad Arensberg helped us understand how communities work and how to work with communities. We are indebted to Kathy Pryzynski, Maureen Groden, and Ken Culp for their thoughtful comments on the earlier editions and to Glenn Blalock and Amanda Peacock for their thoughtful guidance on this, the third edition. We are especially grateful for the contributions of Dolores Shapiro and Michelene Asselin, the original co-authors of *Healthy Places, Healthy People*. Finally, we thank our families, friends, and colleagues for their unrelenting patience and support.

–Lisa Elaine Skemp, PhD, RN, FGSA, FAAN
–Melanie Creagan Dreher, PhD, RN, FAAN
–Susan Primm Lehmann, MSN, RN

ABOUT THE AUTHORS

LISA ELAINE SKEMP, PhD, RN, FGSA, FAAN

Lisa Skemp is Professor and Chair, Department of Health Systems, Leadership, and Policy at Loyola University–Chicago. Skemp taught community health at the University of Iowa College of Nursing and was the Director of the Global Health Initiative at the Iowa Hartford Center of Geriatric Nursing Excellence. Skemp held an Endowed Chair in Gerontological Nursing at Our Lady of the Lake College. In 2000, Skemp received the American Public Health Association New Investigator's Award for her cross-cultural research in the Caribbean, and in 2003 she became a Claire M. Fagin Fellow for her work in rural community healthy aging. After receiving her BSN from Viterbo University, Skemp obtained her master's degree in community health nursing and education and then her doctorate in nursing at the University of Iowa with an emphasis in community capacity building for healthy aging. In 2015, Skemp became a fellow in the Gerontological Society of America and the American Academy of Nursing. Skemp integrates her role as an educator in community health nursing, global health, and gerontology with her research and practice in diverse cultures and communities. Her extensive ethnographic research has included community studies in St. Lucia, the West Indies, rural American Midwest farming communities, Mexican immigrant populations, Sudanese refugee groups, and South India villages. Skemp's contributions to global health include two study-abroad programs in interprofessional community capacity building for healthy aging in St. Lucia and South India.

MELANIE CREAGAN DREHER, PhD, RN, FAAN

Melanie Dreher is the Dean Emeritus of Rush University College of Nursing. An educator for more than 40 years, Dreher has championed nursing as a profession with enormous potential to improve the health and well-being of people in communities. She has taught community assessment, analysis, and intervention at Columbia University, University of Miami, University of Massachusetts, University of Iowa, and Rush University. Dreher earned her bachelor's degree in nursing at Long Island University and her doctorate in anthropology at Columbia

University and Teachers' College. Her extensive ethnographic research in the Caribbean has focused on communities as powerful determinants of the health and welfare of children and adults. As a member of the charter Council of Public Representatives, Dreher brought the realities of people living in communities to the National Institutes of Health. She is a member of the Chicago Board of Health, a trustee at Loyola University–Chicago, and a director on the boards of Trinity Health and Wellmark, Inc., Blue Cross Blue Shield of Iowa and South Dakota. Dreher has received many awards for her contributions to the health of communities, including a citation from the U.S. ambassador for her community development work in Jamaica, where she held a visiting professorship at the University of West Indies. Finally, she has published extensively on culture as an organizing concept in nursing education and practice.

SUSAN PRIMM LEHMANN, MSN, RN

Susan Primm Lehmann received her BSN and MSN from Loyola University Marcella Niehoff School of Nursing in Chicago and has engaged in nursing practice with adult, geriatric, and pediatric populations in acute care and community settings. An Assistant Professor (Clinical) at the University of Iowa College of Nursing, Lehmann has expertise in BSN nursing education focusing on Community and Public Health Nursing (CPHN) with more than 20 years of experience, including BSN curriculum development, mentorship of colleagues new to nursing education, and practicum teaching. She is recognized for her knowledge of and advocacy for the healthcare needs of persons who are homeless, and she has given presentations regionally and nationally on curriculum development for CPHN education. Lehmann is the creator and Director of the Young Community Nurse Clinician Program, an extracurricular mentorship program for talented nursing students who are considering a career in community and public health nursing. Lehmann's areas of research and practice interest include people who experience mental illness in the community, people who are homeless or experience other vulnerabilities, and health promotion across the lifespan. Being an early adopter of the culturally informed community health model of nursing practice, Lehmann is thrilled to be a contributor to this latest edition of *Healthy Places, Healthy People*.

TABLE OF CONTENTS

INTRODUCTION

This is the third edition of a book designed to help students of community/public health nursing learn how to lead change and promote social justice in healthcare locally and globally. Using the concept of culture, they learn how to work *with* residents by first listening to and observing *how communities work and comparing them* to other communities. Then, *with* community partners, students learn to ensure change through programming and public policy. Like the first two editions, this is not your standard textbook. Our goal is not a comprehensive survey of community/public health nursing. Our objective is to guide students in acquiring the *core public health leadership competencies* of community relationship building, inquiry, assessment, analysis, planning, action, evaluation, and persuasion that transcend the categorical public health concerns, such as infectious diseases, maternal-child health, environment monitoring, terrorism, and disaster preparedness. We strive to keep this a small handbook with realistic strategies and practical advice on how to be more effective in mobilizing citizen action for public health. It contains useful tools for preparing, gathering, organizing, and analyzing community information to facilitate work *with* citizens and groups to build capacity for a healthy future and health equity. In many ways, it is a "how-to" book—a public health improvement strategy that can be applied to any community, at any time, to get the jobs of public health and social justice accomplished.

The organizing theme of this edition remains the same: *Healthy places are the building blocks for healthy people.* That means that the capacity of communities to ensure a robust physical and social environment will promote and protect the health of their citizens. In this paradigm, we make the distinction between *creating* health and *treating* health problems—a notion that often is not easily grasped by students who come to their course in public health fresh from the clinical imperatives of the acute care setting. Although access to quality clinical services and illness care is critically important (and disparities in access are symptomatic of an unhealthy community), we do not equate *health* with *healthcare*. It is in the cultural context of the community, stretching well beyond its clinics and hospitals, where the impact of social and environmental determinants is most keenly felt. Obvious examples include clean air, water, and land; safe highways; and uncontaminated food. But they also include the socioeconomic dislocations that place some members of a community on unequal footing—creating local "hot spots" that, left unattended, compromise the health of the whole community.

In this edition, we continue our emphasis on the powerful influence of *place* on health and the role of nurses in leading change. Beginning, perhaps, with the Alameda County study in which human relationships took precedence over health behaviors as the number-one predictor of mortality, research continues to reveal the impact of residential *community culture* on health. In addition to the work of Roberts et al. cited in the first edition (and revisited here), Bender, Clune, & Guruge, 2009; Carolan, Andrews, & Hodnett, 2006; Cummins, Curtis, Diez-Roux, & Macintyre, 2007; Cummins, Stafford, Macintyre, Marmot, & Ellaway, 2005; Drevdahl, 2002; Kerker et al., 2011; Marmot, 2005a and 2005b; Pobutsky, Baker, & Reyes-Salvail, 2015; Stafford & Marmot, 2003; Szwarcwald, da Mota, Damacena, & Pereira, 2011; and Tarlier, Browne, & Johnson, 2007, offer compelling evidence and justification for extending the examination of social and environmental determinants of health beyond the correlation of variables and into the situational realities of community context.

Nursing is defined by *orientation* rather than by *setting*. The nurse who is employed in the cardiology clinic of a tertiary-care setting and who sits on local and national policy boards for cardiac prevention, who speaks to women's groups throughout the community to educate them about the risks for heart disease in women, who establishes self-help programs for women with heart disease, and who links the families of women with cardiac pathology seen in the hospital to community services has a strong *community health orientation*. In contrast, the nurse who is employed in a neighborhood-based prenatal clinic but whose practice is limited to assessing and counseling expectant mothers—ignoring the obvious disparities in birth weight, the burden of parenthood, the lack of day care programs, food and nutrition, transportation to the clinic, and existing regulations and housing policies that compromise the mothers' capacity to raise their children in a healthy and safe environment—may be working in a community setting but does not have a community orientation.

Furthermore, the commonly made distinction between acute care and community care is spurious and diverts our attention from our true mission. Essentially, the presence of a sufficient and well-integrated acute care system falls within the "assurance" responsibility of public health. Hospitals are simply another community institution, not unlike churches, schools, clinics, businesses, and factories, with an important role to play in promoting the health of the public. As public-health providers, our goal is to offer a perspective that prepares *all* students for beginning practice in community health and to fulfill their responsibility for active citizenry. We do not distinguish between "community health nurse" and "public health nurse" and use the term *community/public health nurse* throughout the book.

We continue to use the title *Healthy Places, Healthy People: A Handbook for Culturally Informed Community Nursing Practice* and are delighted to see trends for an increase in the use of "culturally informed" and a decrease in the use of "cultural competence" in the literature. This reinforces the notion that nurses' work *with* communities—each partner bringing unique strengths through *sharing cultural information.*

Healthy People 2020 is referenced heavily. Students then learn how their communities compare with others nationally and that public health is an *interprofessional, community-wide* responsibility. *Healthy People 2020* is guided by two critical questions: (1) *What makes some people healthy and others unhealthy?* and (2) *How can we create a society in which everyone has a chance to live long, healthy lives?* At a time when it is easy to be distracted by categorical problems, initiatives, and funding, we believe effective responses to these two great big societal questions require a comprehensive and unrelenting focus on the health of the *whole* community and its culture.

Healthy People 2020 provides strategies for achieving overarching goals and a project management model, called MAP-IT. With only three categories of interventions and a widely used logic model for planning and implementation, building capacity for community action would seem relatively straightforward. But inspiring communities to take action goes beyond just formulating policies about the sale of cigarettes to minors, educating the public about the dangers of obesity, or cleaning up a polluted river. When we start moving initiatives, such as sex education or improved emission standards, into the *cultural realities* of community life, things get much more complicated. Mobilizing *specific* action with a *specific* community in a specific *place* requires an understanding of the complexities of community culture, with all its diverse citizens, groups, interests, goals, and values.

So what is different about this edition? First of all, no community desires to be "problematized." We contend that community strengths are the "glue" that holds a community together and that it is *within nurses' purview* to discover these strengths. In this edition, a strengths-based assessment is emphasized. We have avoided many references to "vulnerable populations" and "socioeconomic determinants," as such terms suggest a kind of unassailable dependency and weakness that deter us from seeing the opportunities that are waiting to be discovered and activated in a strengths-based, "culturally informed" community health practice.

We took the advice of our readers to better explain how nurses use ethnography and epidemiology to understand the health and the culture of their communities. These concepts are best comprehended not only by explaining what they are and are not but also by emphasizing how they are complementary or "partner" concepts. Beginning in Chapter 1, we juxtapose ethnography and epidemiology and their respective units of analysis—communities and populations—to illustrate the differences and the complementarities between the two scientific orientations in community/public health nursing.

Responding to faculty and student requests, we have added an additional chapter, entitled "The Practice Project." Chapter 4 is a transition chapter that provides practical steps, tools, and activities to help students bridge the concepts from Chapters 1–3 to the applied Chapters 5–6, where they conduct the culturally informed community assessment, and then to Chapters 7–8, where students move into the action and evaluation phases of community/public health nursing.

The passage of the Patient Protection and Affordable Care Act in 2010 has expanded healthcare access to 30 million formerly uninsured Americans and provides unprecedented opportunities for nurses to fulfill their mandate not only to care for the health of the public but also to lead the redesign of healthcare (Glied & Ma, 2015; Institute of Medicine, 2010). Community/public health nurses will lead this change by working with communities to realize their strengths and build the capacity necessary to shape the future of health and healthcare. Finally, we remain committed to the moral imperative for nurses to lead in promoting social justice, equity, and the health of *all* people as enduring values. We embrace the promise of health reform not just for universal *access* to health services but for universal *engagement* in making communities healthy, open environments in which people are welcome to work, play, raise families, and experience long and healthy lives.

–Lisa Skemp, PhD, RN, FGSA, FAAN
–Melanie Dreher, PhD, RN, FAAN
–Susan Lehmann, MSN, RN

1

The Cultural Framework of Community Health

Beginning with *culture* and how it informs nursing practice, this chapter explores the concepts essential to becoming an effective community/public health nurse. It goes on to discuss *communities* and *populations*—two very different but necessary concepts in public health that prompt the need for nurses to incorporate *ethnographic* as well as *epidemiological* inquiries into their practice. The chapter ends with an introduction to the moral imperatives that frame community/public health practice and a discussion of the role of nursing in promoting social justice and leading change in public health.

Chapter 1 Objectives

- Describe the significance of culture as an organizing concept in community/public health nursing practice and the ecological fallacy that has inhibited its application in clinical practice.

- Understand the difference between communities and populations, their usefulness in community/public health practice, and the ways in which they frame public health science.

- Know the difference between equality and equity in ethical community/public health practice and the role of nursing in promoting social justice and leading change in public health.

CULTURALLY INFORMED NURSING PRACTICE

Culture is not a new concept in public health. The importance of knowing a community's culture to determine patterns of illness, health, and the use of health services was documented in the 1950s in a landmark collection titled *Health, Culture, and Community: Case Studies of Public Reactions to Health Programs* (Paul, 1955):

> If you wish to help a community improve its health, you must learn to think like the people.... To assume new health habits, it is wise to ascertain the existing habits, how these habits are linked to one another, what functions they perform, and what they mean to those who practice them. (p. 1)

Nor is culture a new concept for community/public health nurses. More than 60 years ago, George Rosen (1954) advised:

> First and foremost comes a knowledge of the community and its people. This knowledge must be acquired and is just as important for successful public health work as is a knowledge of epidemiology or medicine.... The community/health nurse ... should be consciously aware of the way of life of the people, their goals in life, the motivations that make them do the things they do, [and] the things in life that mean much or little to them. (Rosen, 1954, p. 15)

Using cultural information in practice is a distinguishing feature of the profession of nursing (Dreher, 1996; Leininger, 1988). According to the American Nurses Association (2015):

> Nursing is the protection, promotion, and optimization of health and abilities, prevention of illness and injury, alleviation of suffering through the diagnosis and treatment of human responses, and advocacy in the care of individuals, families, communities, and populations.

Unlike medical practice, in which a streptococcal infection is treated pretty much the same way in Bangkok at it is in London and an appendectomy is fundamentally the same procedure in Kenya as in Canada, nursing practice anticipates and accommodates the wide variation in culturally embedded human *responses* to health, illness, and treatment. To be effective, nurses must know more about their patients than just the biological variables of disease, age, and sex. They must incorporate knowledge of their lifestyles, values, education, occupation, social status, and the ways they interpret illness and treatment.

To improve the health of the public, community nurses need to know more than the rate of HIV infection, the prevalence of diabetes, or the incidence of low-birth-weight babies. They also need to know the community's religious institutions, educational resources, political economy, commonly held values, social norms, and cultural interpretations of health and healthcare. In other words, in public health, just as in personal health services, nurses must use cultural knowledge to inform their practice and optimize the outcomes.

CULTURAL COMPETENCE AND CLINICAL PRACTICE

Culturally competent care has become a mantra of contemporary healthcare practice (Andrews & Boyle, 2008; Betancourt, Green, Carrillo, & Ananeh-Firempong, 2003; Campinha-Bacote & Munoz, 2001; Fahrenwald, Boysen, Fischer, & Maurer, 2001; Leininger, 1988, 1997; University of Kansas, 2015; U.S. Department of Health & Human Services, 2010). According to cultural competence advocates, when care is consistent with traditional beliefs and practices, patients will be more engaged in the plan of care, care will be safer and more appropriate, and clinical outcomes will be improved. Unfortunately, despite nationwide leadership from experts in nursing and medicine, professional organizations, and certifying bodies, routine incorporation of cultural information in patient treatment plans has not been widely achieved (Benkert, Tanner, Guthrie, Oakley, & Pohl, 2005; Fisher, Burnet, Huang, Chin, & Cagney, 2007; Omeri & Malcolm, 2004; Williamson & Harrison, 2010). With the important exception of language translation, most nurses, physicians, and other care providers continue to work in a cultural vacuum when planning the care of their patients, and patient charts seldom include references to cultural information.

These disappointing outcomes do not reflect a lack of will or interest on the part of caregivers but rather a fundamental misunderstanding of culture that leads to confusion and frustration in its application. *Culture* is a social construction that pertains to *groups*. Within any group, some members may embrace all its rules and traditions, while others may embrace only some, and still others may apply them according to the situation. When information that pertains to groups (cultures) is used to make decisions about individuals (patients), an *ecological fallacy* has occurred (Bernard, 2011; Clancy, Berger, & Magliozzi, 2003; Dreher & Mac-Naughton, 2002). To illustrate the ecological fallacy inherent in the application of cultural information in a clinical context, we could use the opposition of the Catholic Church to birth control, based on its ethical religious directives. As an *institution*, the Catholic Church formally opposes birth control, but it is widely known that many Catholics are critical of the directive, support the use of birth control, use or desire to use birth control, and yet still consider themselves devout Catholics.

In the attempt to be culturally sensitive and acknowledge the faiths of our patients, we could wrongly assume that a particular woman of Catholic faith would have no interest in learning about birth control and fail to discuss the range of options available to her. This would be a misapplication of cultural knowledge. Just knowing a patient's ethnicity, national origin, or religion is not sufficient to inform care. Achieving cultural competence in a *clinical* practice requires soliciting each patient's interpretation of his or her illness episode and expectation of treatment by asking the right questions and listening carefully to the responses, which must then be included and implemented in a culturally informed plan of care (Kleinman, 1980). Cultures are *not* monolithic and unchanging, and patients are *not* frozen in cultural traditions, unable to modify their behavior or learn new ways.

Although the cultural competence movement emerged and accelerated in response to an increasingly multiethnic, global society, understanding health and illness from the perspective of the patient is not a new concept. It is, in fact, the foundation for *patient-centered care*. The goal of the cultural competence movement was to prepare us for an increasingly diverse world, but it also raised our sensitivity to the cultural factors that affect the care of *all* patients and that likely were taken for granted when patients and providers looked much more alike. Real culture-informed practice begins with acknowledging that *all* patients (not just those of a different ethnicity, national origin, or language group) are influenced by their cultures and deserve *culturally informed* courses of treatment. And further, patients *and* providers bring "cultural baggage," of·which they are likely to be unaware, to every healthcare encounter.

CULTURAL CAPITAL AND PUBLIC HEALTH

In public health practice, culture is a potent and highly applicable concept. Because information about groups (cultures) (Edelson, 2008; Fahrenwald et al., 2001; Kreuter & McClure, 2004; Racher & Annis, 2007) is used to understand and manage the health of groups (communities and populations), an ecological fallacy does not occur. The most successful public health initiatives and community-based programs target culturally relevant community groups, engage community leaders, work with and through local institutions, and establish culturally prescribed channels of communication (Tripp-Reimer, Choi, Skemp Kelley, & Enslein, 2001). This *culturally informed* approach to public health begins with an inquiry and analysis of (a) how and why a particular public health problem is embedded in the *cultural context* of community life, and (b) the *cultural capital* available to fix it. Cultural capital is the arsenal of community institutions, leaders, customs, knowledge, and values that can be invested to promote healthy communities and the well-being of all their citizens (Hopkins & Mehanna, 2000, 2003).

The recent epidemic of childhood obesity provides a useful example of the potential of cultural information to inform community/public health practice. As a serious public health problem with a significant impact on community resources over time, childhood obesity is more than an individual nutritional problem or eating disorder to be treated in a clinical setting. Examining childhood obesity in the context of community life reveals the cultural norms, values, and behaviors that pertain to physical activity, body-image preferences, parent-child relationships, and food preparation and consumption. It expands the breadth and depth of interventions and enlists the community's cultural capital (e.g., teachers, coaches, local athletes, grocers, fast-food restaurants, parks and playgrounds, churches, grandmothers, schools, grocery stores, policymakers, and community celebrations) to increase the effectiveness of the intervention and reduce the costs. Cultural information about where, when, and what children eat and the social meaning of food consumption both for children and caregivers provide guidance for social marketing, public education, community coalitions, and the organization of system-level services.

This approach to the resolution of a public health epidemic of a personal health problem stands in marked contrast to the usual "deficit" analysis of a community's health, focused almost exclusively on what is "wrong" with communities—what they lack or need to become healthy places that will generate healthy populations. Creating healthy communities by investing in actual and potential cultural capital lessens the reliance on expensive clinical resources needed for treating each child separately and focuses on more enduring and far-reaching changes in society and the built environment to ameliorate and prevent the epidemic level of childhood obesity in the community. Mobilizing community strengths around a public health issue also models community self-determination and self-help that can be mobilized for other human service problems ranging from traffic safety and clean air and water to HIV/AIDS and elder support.

CULTURAL BARRIERS? NOT REALLY

It is never acceptable to cite a patient's "culture" as the reason a provider's care plan has not been followed, and it is *equally* unacceptable to attribute the lack of success in public health initiatives to "culture barriers" rooted in the community. Such outcomes almost always reflect the difficulties and frustrations encountered by the public health team in effectively acquiring and interpreting the community's cultural perspective and adjusting the plan of care accordingly. This process requires practice and patience, and it is not uncommon for providers of the dominant group to assume that cultural barriers are minimized and partnerships for community action are optimized only when healthcare providers and community residents are of the same ethnic and language groups. Although having greater diversity in the provider community is highly desirable, ample evidence suggests that cultural barriers in clinical and public health practice are attributable not so much to the lack of community-provider sameness as they are to the failure of providers to establish meaningful relationships with persons and groups (Epps, Skemp, & Specht, 2015). Knowing the community, its people, and its culture is the responsibility of *all* members of the healthcare team—not just those who bear cultural similarities to community members. Cultural understanding is the key to effective provider-community relationships, without which it is impossible to formulate and execute a healthy community agenda (Drevdahl, 1995).

In the H1N1 flu epidemic of 2010, when it was important first to immunize those most at risk (children and pregnant women), health departments did not have to go from house to house to ensure that immunizations were carried out effectively and efficiently. Instead, they deployed the communities' cultural capital (radio, newspapers, Internet, primary schools, faith institutions, after-school programs, neighborhood pharmacies, city colleges, hospital emergency rooms, teachers, volunteers, obstetricians, and primary-care physicians) to ensure that women and children would be protected first.

During the African Ebola crisis of 2014, conventional means of communication (newspapers, TV, and radio) were used to disseminate accurate information about the virus in rural and isolated areas. In densely populated cities, where more educated persons had access to cell phones and the Internet, social media was an effective means of acquiring and sharing health information. Social media users were recognized as some of the most influential people in society who helped spread the word about the dangers of Ebola (Putic, 2014).

COMMUNITIES AND POPULATIONS: PARTNER CONCEPTS

The terms *community* and *population* often are used interchangeably in public health practice. They are interrelated but different in important ways that make them effective "partner concepts" in advancing the health of the public.

COMMUNITIES

In its broadest use, the term *community* can be applied to almost any configuration of people whose values, characteristics, and/or interests unite them in some way (for example, a religious community, a retirement community, or a university community). In public health practice, we ordinarily define community as the unit in which the cultural impact on health and illness is most observable: a place (environment) where people (populations) live and interact with each other in routine and predictable ways (social organization). But communities are not just collections of people occupying the same space at the same time. Rather, they are composed of institutions (religion, commerce, government, music, recreation, art and architecture, education, domestic patterns) and regular cycles of human activity that bring people together in socially organized ways to learn, work, play, and participate in family activities. Community members may attend the same schools, work for the same employers, live in the same apartment buildings, or exercise at the same gyms. It is not necessary for all members of the community to know all the other members of the community or to hold the same beliefs, share the same values, or engage in the same behavior, but ordinarily, overarching community values and rules and sets of exchanges—formal and informal—guide the ways in which community residents behave and interact with one another.

As the keepers of culture, communities have lives of their own. Individuals may enter and leave a community over time with varying degrees of impact—if any—on its culture. On the other hand, communities and the cultures that perpetuate them are not static. They are constantly refreshed (and disrupted) by new persons, new knowledge, and new circumstances. Although we tend to think of communities as harmonious places, guided by established cultural rules, their dynamic nature makes conflict inevitable as traditional values are challenged. The presence of conflict within a community is a normal vehicle for culture change and, although it can be unsettling, does not necessarily challenge the integrity of the community.

Finally, a community is defined from the inside—a continuing saga, a society with a history and a future, constantly changing the way in which it uses "place" (time and space) and is being changed by it. Some communities look very much like they did 50 years ago, while others have changed dramatically. In the late 19th century, American communities grew and flourished at each stop of a burgeoning railway system, creating residential areas and "downtown" centers. With the introduction of automobile transportation in the 1920s, however, families moved to new and larger homes on the outskirts of towns, creating suburbs. Schools, hospitals, and businesses followed. Shopping centers replaced the small shops and services that had once served to bring people together in villages and town centers. These transformative changes in where and how people live, work, and play are simultaneously the genesis and the outcome of human communities over time. Today, the Internet and social media have created virtual interactions, transactions, and communities, heralding an unparalleled global interconnectivity among humans that transcends their physical environments. But even residential communities are a *subjective reality*, with no designated geo-political boundaries and often defined differently by members of the same community.

POPULATIONS

Populations, in comparison to communities, are somewhat easier to comprehend, because they are *objective realities*, exactly equal to the sum of their parts. Broadly defined, a population is simply a category of humans that has at least one characteristic in common (e.g., residence, eye color, religion, etc.). Traditionally, however, we think of populations as the number of people who reside in a specific geo-political unit at a specific time (e.g., the population of Louisiana in 2015 or the population of Franklin County in 2012). This practical definition is consistent with the goals of public health *administration*. It reflects the responsibilities of boards of health or health departments to make rules that promote and protect the health and safety of the people of a corresponding geo-political unit (e.g., municipality, incorporated village, county, state, country, etc.) through the enactment of laws and policies. Examples include regulations prohibiting smoking in public places and car-seat laws to protect infants and small children. Populations also are important in public health *research* as the units of analysis we examine and correlate statistically to identify health risks (e.g., the population of cigarette smokers is "at risk" for lung cancer, children living in old homes or on busy streets are at greater risk for lead poisoning). When categories of persons within a community are singled out for a public health intervention and/or research, they often are referred to as *target populations*.

Populations are snapshots of a category of people in a specific place at a specific time, taken from the outside, for specific and important purposes—the administration of services or medical research. They do not constitute a group in which members necessarily interact with each other. There is no reason, for example, for all the persons diagnosed with asthma in the city of Spokane to know each other and convene socially. On the other hand, if nurse practitioners determine that their patients with asthma have much to gain from each other and decide to bring them together for learning and mutual support, they are potentially transforming a health population into a therapeutic community, which has a life of its own. The size and characteristics of populations change as individuals are born, die, or migrate in or out of an area. From 2000 to 2013, for example, the ethnic composition of the population of Cloudcroft, New Mexico, first saw an increase in the Hispanic or Latino composition and then a decrease in Hispanic or Latino composition from 15.5% to 10.3% of the population (City-Data.com, n.d.). The community of Cloudcroft, however, has continued to exist, incorporating these changes in ethnic composition within its ever-changing community culture.

Although population and community are not the same, they are related in important ways in public health practice. All communities have constituent populations, but not all populations have or are communities. Sometimes, populations and communities are conterminous. In the tiny village of Shelburne Falls, Massachusetts, for example, the population and the community are composed of the same people, all of whom benefit from the services provided by the Town of Shelburne Board of Health. When a family moves away from Shelburne Falls, it alters the population, but its departure may or may not affect the community, depending on the role and position of that family in community life. Even a small place like Shelburne Falls contains several populations—elders, schoolchildren, persons with diabetes, business owners, Baptists—and some of these categories may create sub-communities that extend beyond the borders of Shelburne Falls. In comparison, the very large municipality of Chicago has a population of roughly 3 million people, organized into 50 geo-political subpopulations (districts or wards). It also contains at least 77 neighborhoods, more or less defined by residents and businesses that occupy them. The geo-political districts and the neighborhood communities composing Chicago must all be considered to provide comprehensive, culturally informed public health services. Populations are critical for ensuring the distribution of health services and management of epidemics, but ultimately, people do not live out their lives in populations; they live out their lives in communities, where health and illness are created and managed. Communities are the lens through which we identify cultural capital (including district administration) that has the potential to improve the health of the public beyond what medicine alone can accomplish.

ETHNOGRAPHY AND EPIDEMIOLOGY

The important relationship between community and population in public health practice is reflected in its two major modes of inquiry: ethnography and epidemiology.

Ethnographic research examines *whole communities* to comprehend the constellation of local conditions in which health and illness are embedded. Ethnography, derived from the social sciences (particularly anthropology), seeks to understand the impact of community culture on health and healthcare and to identify public health improvements in the social, economic, and political domains of community life.

Epidemiological research, in contrast, explores variations in the patterns, causes, and effects of disease and disability in *specified populations*, using statistical correlations to identify probable causes. Although its origins are in medical science, epidemiology has exceeded the contributions of clinical medicine for improving the health of the public by identifying "risk factors" and creating opportunities for disease prevention and early detection.

As cornerstones of public health inquiry, epidemiology and ethnography acknowledge the mounting evidence of the relationship between health status and social status. In response, epidemiologists have expanded the usual biological risk factors (age, sex, and race) to include social and economic variables, such as occupation, income, education, and, most recently, ethnicity (often, inappropriately, used as a proxy for culture). Statistical studies of ethnic populations have yielded important correlations between disease and ethnicity that serve to alert healthcare providers to the need to manage risk: African Americans, for example, are at risk for hypertension; American Indians are at risk for diabetes. Although correlations between disease and ethnicity are useful for alerting clinicians to potential risk, they alone cannot explain how identified risk factors are connected in the complex neighborhoods, villages, and cities where people live out their daily lives. Why, for example, do some American Indians develop diabetes while others do not? Or, why do some African Americans have high blood pressure while others do not? Why is the death rate rising in middle-age American Caucasians and decreasing in other ethnic groups (Case & Deaton, 2015)? In contrast to the epidemiologists' focus on populations, ethnographers examine culture not as an individual risk factor (ethnicity) but as "the matrix of collective influences that shape the lives of groups and individuals" (Corin, 1994, p. 101). They see health inequalities rooted in community culture, where the conditions and causes of disparities are most evident and where health is situated in the social and economic disruptions of community life (Cummins, Curtis, Diez-Roux, & Macintyre, 2007; Cummins, Stafford, Macintyre, Marmot, & Ellaway, 2005; Marmot, 2005a).

Public health practice is well served by the complementarity of these two scientific traditions. When epidemiological studies and bio-statistical data on health disparities are reexamined in the light of ethnographic studies of single communities, it creates an understanding of "situated risk" and opportunities for solutions. As a result, we have an increasingly better understanding of the significance of communities for growing and sustaining healthy populations. Reducing the incidence of lung cancer would be comparatively easy if the knowledge that tobacco inhalation and lung cancer are highly correlated were a sufficient disincentive for people to stop smoking cigarettes. But the "logic" of healthy behavior is mitigated by psychological and social pleasures, the political strength of the tobacco industry, the economic impact on tobacco growers and vendors, state and municipal revenue

streams from cigarette taxation, and, most recently, the glamour marketing of fla-
vored tobacco and e-cigarettes to adolescents, young adults, and specific ethnic
groups.

> At the time of this writing, our smallest state, Rhode Island, has the third
> highest tax on cigarettes, at $3.50 per pack. If public health efforts were
> able to set and reach a public health goal of reducing the number of Rhode
> Island cigarette-smokers by 50,000, assuming the average smoker con-
> sumes one pack per day, the state would stand to lose $63,875,000 in
> annual revenues that support healthcare, education, and highway improve-
> ments. Looking at state-local tax rates, the highest is $6.16 in Chicago,
> Illinois (Boonn, 2015).

MORAL IMPERATIVES OF HEALTH AND NURSING

Health as a continuously changing relationship between the environment and
population, mitigated by community culture, is easily grasped when common
public health problems of the past, such as scurvy and smallpox, are compared
with contemporary problems, such as chronic illness, obesity, motor-vehicle accidents, drug abuse, gun violence, nuclear disaster, terrorism, and HIV/AIDS. In
Healthy People 2020, 13 new foci were added to the list of achievable objectives,
demonstrating increased public concern about the under-represented populations
of children and adolescents; older adults; and lesbian, gay, bisexual, and transgender people. Additional new topics included social determinants of health, global
health, disaster preparedness, health-related quality of life and well-being, blood
disorders and blood safety, genetics, dementia, sleep health, and healthcare-associated infections.

THE HEALTH OF POPULATIONS

Given the dynamic definition of health as always being in flux and constantly
adapting to a changing environment, how do we evaluate the health of our

communities? It is tempting to measure the health of a community by simply aver-aging the personal health indicators of the members composing its constituent population. In the recently formulated *population health* enterprise, for instance, the goal is to organize care in a way that improves the health of a designated pop-ulation, producing better clinical outcomes at a reduced cost. Success is indicated by reductions in disease or disability as well as in the more appropriate and cost-effective use of services by the category of persons being managed.

Population health requires clinicians to go beyond seeing each patient as a single unit of care and to identify problems that may underlie the treatment of many or all persons in a specific category—whether a shared medical diagnosis, age group, residence in the same neighborhood, or behavioral health problem. Providers look for ways to address the problem more efficiently or to prevent it from occurring altogether. Incentivized by payer-sponsored (commercial and public) risk-sharing opportunities to produce better outcomes at a reduced cost, population health providers depart from the individual patient orientation of traditional clinical practice. In the sense that it engages and supports community-based prevention and health promotion activities, such as healthy school lunches, elder transporta-tion, tobacco policies, centered pregnancy care, and changes in the environment to promote safety and exercise, population health often complements the classic efforts of public health agencies by addressing a broader range of influential fac-tors, such as the built environment or healthier workplaces. Nevertheless, its suc-cess is determined solely by the health of designated populations and their collec-tive use of health services (for example, using nurse practitioners to decrease ER visits for common ailments, such as colds and ear infections, in uninsured or underinsured school-age children).

MEASURING EQUITY

Although population health has received significant attention as a strategy for improving clinical outcomes, only one of the overarching goals of *Healthy People 2020* specifically addressed disease, disability, and injury in levels of populations:

- **To attain high-quality, longer lives free of preventable disease, disability, injury, and premature death**

The remaining three goals addressed quality of life, health promotion, and social and physical environments that support good health "for *all*":

- **To achieve health equity, eliminate disparities, and improve the health of all groups**

- **To create social and physical environments that promote good health for all**

- **To promote quality of life, healthy development, and healthy behaviors across all life stages**

The references to "all," "all groups," and "all life stages" are significant. They imply that the health of a town or city cannot be determined by averaging the health of citizens across neighborhoods and acknowledge that the presence of inequalities or disparities in even *one* urban neighborhood puts the health of *all* urban neighborhoods at risk. *Health disparities or inequalities* refer to health conditions or outcomes that are associated with some form of disadvantage. In *Healthy People 2010*, the elimination of health disparities was one of only two overarching goals. *Healthy People 2020* took the health-disparity goal to the new level of *achieving health equity*:

> Attainment of the highest level of health for all people. Achieving health equity requires valuing everyone equally with focused and ongoing societal efforts to address avoidable inequalities, historical and contemporary injustices, and the elimination of health and healthcare disparities. (U.S. Department of Health & Human Services, Office of Minority Health, 2010)

This revised goal reflected a subtle but profound shift from measuring the health of a community by the presence or absence of disease and disability to measuring the health of a community by the presence or absence of disparities. In so doing, it fully acknowledged the impact of social and economic marginality on health and healthcare and introduced the concepts of equity and equality.

The goal of public health practice is system-level intervention that goes beyond remedying a particular *inequality* by building the community's capacity to address health *equity*. Although the terms are often used interchangeably, equality and equity are different in important ways. *Equality* is a fundamental value in American culture, based on the notion that all humans are created equal, have the right to participate in society equally (one person: one vote), and should have equal access to the same societal resources—education, protection, freedom of religion, transportation infrastructure, healthcare, and so forth. *Equity* introduces the notion of *social justice*, indicating that although opportunities may be equally offered, we live in a society in which some members—by virtue of racism, sexism, poverty, home life, or other factors—are impeded from accessing these opportunities.

For example, a city health department provides free mammography for all adult female residents, but some women are unable to access this service because of work schedules, transportation issues, or family responsibilities. A just society ensures the resources necessary to create a level playing field and reduces impediments to accessing it. Without equality *and* social justice, there can be no fairness in healthcare.

COMMUNITY/PUBLIC HEALTH AND NURSES' CALL TO ACTION

Nurses' awareness of the socioeconomic dislocations in health emerged at the turn of the 20th century, when they began to note differences in the customs and health patterns of the immigrant communities whom they served. Visiting homes of tenement families and staffing prenatal and child health clinics, nurses became familiar with the social and economic inequities that kept these neighborhoods on uneven footing, creating disparities in health and healthcare. Notwithstanding the brilliant and courageous activism of nurse leaders, such as Lillian Wald, the founder of public health nursing in the United States, the role of nurses typically was limited to supervising home care and clinic visits and encouraging individuals and families to adopt healthy behaviors.

For the most part, they were unable to engage in the public action required to address the myriad of daily assaults on health experienced by families with whom they worked. Even as passionate advocates, without the theoretical understanding and practical experience of working at the system level, they were no match for the powerful social and economic forces that perpetuated disparities in health and access to care and allowed the conditions of poor public health to exist (Dreher, 1982a; Dreher & MacNaughton, 2002; Drevdahl, 1995, 2002; Fahrenwald, Taylor, Kneipp, & Canales, 2007; Tripp-Reimer, Skemp Kelley, & Enslein, 2001).

Now, a century later, the nursing profession has experienced two major calls to action. First, the Affordable Care Act (ACA) identified a compelling need for advanced practice nurses to ensure quality care for aging and chronically ill populations, including those with behavioral and mental health problems.

And just months following passage of the act, the Institute of Medicine (IOM) published *The Future of Nursing: Leading Change, Advancing Health*. Similar to the ACA, it recommended radical increases in the number of advanced practice registered nurses (APRNs), but, most important, it also challenged the nursing profession to *lead the redesign of healthcare*. A culturally informed practice that engages civic society improves quality, reduces costs, and increases access through community-based care and helps in the redesign of healthcare by understanding people's lives.

Six decades of understanding people's lives—as previewed from the beginning of this chapter to the end—are the unique and essential contribution nurses bring to the care equation; this span of time is the foundation for an effective and moral public health practice. With an emerging arsenal of theories and experiences that recognize whole communities as fundamental units of public health service, nurses are increasingly equipped to take group-level action. They now have the requisite skill set and experience to intervene at the system level and foster relationships that build and sustain trust to generate "culturally transformative" (Tripp-Reimer, Skemp Kelley, & Enslein, 2001), far-reaching reform that will achieve health equity. The IOM report and the ACA are calling on nurses to embrace the "big patients" of whole communities and enter the public and political arena in partnership with community groups. Kathleen Chafey's plea in 1996 is as cogent today as it was 20 years ago:

> Nurses must care about what happens to *groups* [sic] of citizens,
> as well as particular clients.... Although proponents of "caring"

seem to have drawn a distinction between an ethic of justice and an ethic of care, this is bipolar, even antithetical. Building the health of communities requires universal application of the principles of justice. It further requires that nurses care enough about their communities and the individuals in them to do battle in political, social, and economic arenas. (Chafey, 1996, p. 15)

Nurses have been liberated to go beyond assessment of the community as just providing the context of patient care to advancing the community itself as the *object* of care, taking action to ensure equity and social justice (Butterfield, 1990, 2002; Dreher, 1982a; Dreher & MacNaughton, 2002; Drevdahl, 1995; Fahrenwald, Taylor, Kneipp, & Canales, 2007) as well as the fair distribution of health resources (Levy & Sidel, 2006). Grounded in principles of community self-determination, a brilliant and timeless example of what nurses can do when they focus on creating healthy communities is presented in *9226 Kercheval Street* (Milio, 1970). While working as a young visiting nurse in an inner-city community in Detroit, Michigan, Milio discovered the most effective assistance she could provide to the mothers on public assistance was to help them be independent wage earners. To do this, she partnered with those mothers to establish a cooperative daycare center where they could safely leave their children while they entered the workforce. Fighting many political and financial battles, Milio helped her clients to initiate a daycare center and run it independently. Fundamentally, she engaged citizens in community-level action in which they identified and deployed community cultural capital to create a healthier, more wholesome environment for children and their mothers. And at the end of the catastrophic Detroit riots, the Moms and Tots Center was the only building left standing.

Healthy Places, Healthy People is designed to prepare students and nurses to work with whole communities, to take system-level action, and to help communities build the capacity to ensure healthcare for all citizens (Fahrenwald et al., 2007). It is based on three premises:

■ Health is a basic human right of all persons.

■ Healthy places are the starting point for healthy people.

■ Community/public health nurses are accountable for system-level action to build community capacity and to ensure social justice for health and healthcare.

2

CULTURALLY INFORMED COMMUNITY HEALTH PRACTICE

A culturally informed approach for working with communities requires a different way of thinking and a different set of skills than clinical nursing practice. This chapter introduces community/public health nursing practice, exploring its distinctive features and explaining its guiding concepts, units of intervention, methods of assessment and action, nurse-client relationships, and guiding values.

CHAPTER 2 OBJECTIVES

- Within a historical context, identify the goals and unique features of community/public health nursing.

- Explain how community and population work together as guiding concepts in community/public health nursing.

- Specify the advantages of a community health paradigm as opposed to a clinical paradigm.

- Understand the distinctive features of the nurse-community relationship.

- Describe the assumptions, ethics, and values of public health practice.

WHAT IS COMMUNITY/PUBLIC HEALTH NURSING?

Community/public health nursing differs from other kinds of practice in two important ways:

- The unit of practice is the whole community—the physical and social environment, the people, and their social organizations.

- The objective of practice is to promote and protect the health of the public.

These two features—communities as clients and the emphasis on health—are related in important ways. Creating health, as opposed to just treating disease, requires community-level intervention in which healthy places are the foundation for healthy people.

THE COMMUNITY HEALTH LEGACY

The tradition for community/public health nursing was established in Liverpool, England, during the Victorian age, with the support of William Rathbone, a wealthy merchant and social reformer. On the advice of Florence Nightingale, Rathbone opened a training school in 1862 to prepare district nurses to oversee the health of designated communities. Meanwhile, American nursing activists, with the assistance of prominent women who had been to England and were strongly influenced by the work of Rathbone and Nightingale, began to institute district nursing in the United States. By the time Lillian Wald, the founder of public health nursing in the United States, established the Henry Street Settlement in New York City in the 1890s (Feld, 2008; Henry Street Settlement, n.d.; Wald, 1915), district-nursing organizations already had been established in several American cities.

These community health services, modeled after those in Great Britain, were available to the entire population in a designated area. A young Wald acknowledged the importance of prevention as she practiced nursing in the immigrant Jewish communities. Similar to what anthropologists do using ethnographic methods, she chose to live in the community she served to better understand its challenges and assets from the perspective of its citizens. She contended that all people, whether sick or well, should receive health services (Buhler-Wilkerson, 1993). Starting as a volunteer, she and her colleagues educated residents in the Lower East Side of New York City about how diseases were transmitted and how to control infection. In her book *Windows on Henry Street* (1934), Wald explained:

> Our experience in one small East Side section, a block perhaps, had led to a next contact, and a next, in widening circles, until our community relationships have come to include the city, the state, the national government, and the world at large. (p. 167)

In addition to establishing a visiting nurse service, Wald established a school nurse program to attend to the health needs of school-age children and their families, and she eventually introduced housing, education, employment assistance, and community recreational programs. Wald understood that the fundamental changes required to improve the health and welfare of poor immigrants could not be accomplished by a visiting program alone. She lobbied for health inspections of the workplace and for on-site health professionals to protect workers from unsafe conditions; she persuaded President Theodore Roosevelt to create a Federal Children's Bureau; and she convinced the New York Board of Education to hire its first nurse. In 1912, Wald helped found the National Organization for Public Health Nursing and served as its first president.

Following these early examples scattered throughout the major cities of the United States, district nursing also was brought to rural areas, mainly through the efforts of voluntary organizations, such as the American Red Cross. Universal service to the entire community was the hallmark of district nursing. After the turn of the 20th century, however, there was a marked shift toward specialization in public health nursing. This was prompted by a trend toward disease-oriented categorical funding programs, such as tuberculosis control and management of sexually transmitted infections. Formerly generalists, district nurses took on specialized roles in the care of individuals with particular health problems. With the exception of rural areas, universal service was gradually relinquished and replaced by an increasing concentration on *categorical* programs, such as programs to control communicable disease, and on special populations, such as pregnant women.

With the passage of Medicare funding in 1965, even rural communities were convinced to give up the comprehensive health promotion services of district nurses and replace them with illness care for specific individuals provided by home health nurses from a centralized visiting nurse association (Dreher, 1984). Whether community/public health nurses should be generalists, providing comprehensive services to the whole community, or specialists, providing illness care to individuals at home, has been debated for many decades. According to the Quad Council of Public Health Nursing Organizations (2004), there are two levels of community/public health competencies: the staff nurse generalist and the manager/specialist/consultant.

As our healthcare system incorporates the Affordable Care Act (ACA), it is contributing to a cultural shift back to the original spirit of health promotion and the prevention of disease. It is anticipated that healthcare funds will continue to increase as an investment in health promotion, disease prevention, and primary care to meet the needs of formerly uninsured persons and communities across the nation. For example, through expansion of community health centers, it is estimated that around 21.3 million persons will be served by 2014, up 4.3 million from 2011 (Whitehouse.gov, 2012).

THE COMMUNITY PRACTICE PARADIGM

Caring for a whole community requires thinking about nursing in a different way. To better understand community/public health nursing, it is useful to compare the practice of nurses engaged in the care of whole communities to promote public health with that of nurse clinicians engaged in the care of individuals and families to prevent and manage illness.

COMMUNITY CLIENTS

Focusing on the health of a whole town, county, or city neighborhood clearly distinguishes public health from clinical practice, but is the client a population or a community? In Chapter 1, "The Cultural Framework of Community Health," we learned that populations and communities are *complementary* perspectives for monitoring and protecting the health of the public.

Unlike populations, communities are not concrete or defined by external parameters, such as political boundaries or disease categories. As we learned earlier, they are subjectively defined from the inside. The same residentially based population, for example, could be described as a single community by a local politician, as two communities by teachers working in its two school districts, or as several communities by members of various ethnic subpopulations. Geo-politically based health departments are most effective when they combine epidemiological data on populations with an understanding of the cultural matrix of health and illness in the communities they serve and the cultural capital available to address it.

Suggested Activity

Using the definitions of community and population in Chapter 1, identify populations within your community, and name possible communities within these populations.

COMMUNITY PRACTICE GOALS

Ultimately, the goal of public health practice is a healthy community. But what is a healthy community? The measure of a community's health is not simply the aggregate of the health status of its individual citizens, nor is it found only in its most affluent neighborhoods. To determine the health of a community, we must look to its poorest areas, where unsafe housing, dangerous streets, substandard schools, underemployment, lack of access, and lack of voice are symptoms of social and economic inequities that affect the health and safety of the entire community. The cultural capital of a community to address inequities and disparities in health comes from citizens and institutions within all sectors of the community. A healthy community is a physical, economic, and cultural infrastructure that has the potential to fulfill the overarching goals of *Healthy People 2020*.

One of the objectives of *Healthy People 2020* is to increase the proportion of adolescents who have had a wellness checkup in the past 12 months to 75.6%. To do this effectively, population data *and* community cultural data are required. It is important to know, at the very least, the size of the adolescent population, family type, insurance status, and the number of persons who have had wellness checkups to determine whether the goal has been achieved. To make the program effective, however, it is important to know the role and status of adolescents in the specified communities and where they fit in community life (that is, where they live, where and when they get together, how often, and for what purposes). With this information, community health teams can be more useful and efficient by incorporating the places in which adolescents in the community already routinely come together— for example, schools and recreation centers. Such cultural knowledge reduces the costs of launching programs, increases participation, and promotes sustainability.

Building Community Capacity

In clinical practice, nurses are responsible for working directly with their patients and families to manage personal health problems. In public health, an essential community/public nursing responsibility is to enhance the community's capacity to create or extend a healthy community agenda and to protect and promote the health of citizens now and in the future. *Community capacity* is the strength and ability of local groups and institutions to manage the various changes, difficulties, and opportunities that will occur over the decades. Although many situations and trends are not within their control, the healthiest communities have plans for mobilizing material and social resources to manage adverse events and to protect the growth and sustainability of community life. Every community, including those with limited resources, has cultural capital that has the potential to be leveraged to create a healthy, or healthier, community.

In some respects, building community capacity is not unlike helping individuals and families acquire the skills and resilience to successfully manage the problems, losses, crises, and adjustments that occur over a lifetime. In community practice, however, nurses build capacity by identifying and mobilizing community cultural capital and working through and with community leaders, institutions, and groups to create a healthy community agenda for achieving a sustainable future. In places that have an active citizen infrastructure with a demonstrated capacity for community development and social planning, residents have the best chance for reaching a satisfactory resolution of health and social problems.

Cultural Capital

To better understand community cultural capital, consider a scenario in which the vision and hearing statuses of children between the ages of 10 and 14 are to be screened. It is neither necessary nor practical to send each child to an audiologist or optician to be properly assessed, nor would it be particularly effective to announce the availability of a screening program and just hope that parents and children would show up. Instead, the program can be designed and organized through the school system, where most children are conveniently gathered at pre-dictable times. In addition, school records can be used to identify those children who are absent during screening and require follow-up to ensure the evaluation of the entire targeted population. Because schools are part of the community's cultural capital, such programs can be scheduled routinely each year so that every child's performance can be traced over time at regular intervals. Finally, through community action at the policy level, such programs could be funded and bud-geted as part of an ongoing responsibility shared by the school systems and the public health department to monitor the vision and hearing statuses of children annually.

Although this example of schools as cultural capital may seem exceptionally obvi-ous, it is important to understand that each community has distinct characteris-tics that must be systematically and compre-hensively identified and analyzed, incorporated into an inventory of community cultural capital, and mobilized, as necessary, through culture-specific action. Thus, parent-child community health practice is not just about providing personal health services in the form of prenatal care to a target population of high-risk mothers in prenatal clinics. Rather, it is

Suggested Activity

Identify three examples of cultural capital in your community, and consider how they can be lever-aged for the health and well-being of the community.

about identifying and creating community resources available to meet the needs of childbearing families in the community—currently *and* in the future. As discussed in Chapter 1, the community is greater than the sum of its parts and offers more opportunities for intervention than any single member could provide.

COMMUNITY ASSESSMENT

Just as clinical practice begins with a systematic assessment of the individual client, community/public health nursing begins and continues to be informed by an ongoing comprehensive analysis of the community client and its health issues, concerns, strengths, and expectations (American Nurses Association, 2007). On entering the examining room, the clinician's first view of the patient includes a systematic head-to-toe assessment. Similarly, community/public health nurses *systematically* assess a community by observing the neighborhood, town, city, or county and identifying major highways, commercial centers, schools, factories, government buildings, parks, perhaps a mountain range or prairie, a river dividing commercial areas, a residential suburb, recreational areas, and urban centers easing into farmland.

Whereas the clinician interviews the patient, determining his or her age, ethnicity, residence, religion, occupation, and educational level, the community/public health nurse determines the socio-demographic characteristics of the population—age distribution, educational level, religions, occupations, ethnic groups, and so on. Clinicians explore the physical and behavioral aspects of their patients and how they function, but community/public health nurses evaluate the community's social and economic institutions, class structures, neighborhood associations and government, and the ways in which they relate in a specific environment. In personal health services, health statuses and health deviations are identified objectively through such techniques as physical examinations and laboratory tests, and they are evaluated subjectively by taking histories and ascertaining the clients' perspectives on their health problems. Objective and subjective findings are included in the analysis and diagnosis. Similarly, in community health practice, inferences are drawn from subjective and objective sources to determine demographic, sociological, environmental, and economic data, as well as from health status and health-utilization data.

Assessment tools used in the community include reviews of epidemiological studies, air and water pollution indicators, measures of health disparities, socio-demographic statistics, and possibly community-based and household studies. In addition to quantitative information, community data include local definitions, how community members are related, and the prevailing values related to health and illness. These can be obtained directly by talking with community members, key informants, and stakeholders and by attending community events. Additionally, culture-related data can be obtained from community websites and media sources, including social media, radio, television, and local newspapers, and from observations of public behavior and community life.

When populations and communities are the primary units of nursing intervention, it is common to think in terms of rates, patterns, and trends when describing actual and potential health problems. For example, an individual patient either has or does not have heart disease, but a population has a *rate* of heart disease that may compare favorably or unfavorably with the rate of heart disease in another population in the community or with a previous time period for the same population. In clinical practice, a woman is either pregnant or not, but in community/public health nursing, it is possible for a community to be "a little bit" pregnant or "a lot" pregnant. Paired with descriptive data about the community, statistical population data are the direct observations and "lab results" that help diagnose the health of populations and determine a community's health risks. An analysis of the dynamic and synergistic interplay of the environment, the population, and the social organization reveals the cultural capital as well as the health risks of a community and provides the basis for designing a healthy community agenda.

COMMUNITY PLANNING AND INTERVENTION: THE FUTURE ORIENTATION OF COMMUNITY/PUBLIC HEALTH NURSING

Clinicians work with patients to determine the healthcare goals and treatment strategies that make up a care plan. Similarly, community/public health nurses—in partnership with the community—use assessment data to identify and prioritize the health-risk profile of the community and the cultural capital that informs a healthy community agenda. But unlike a patient care plan, comprehensive planning for the community's health is not something that is undertaken and completed within a specific health event, beginning with assessment and ending in evaluation. In fact, the timing and sequencing of public health practice is one of its most distinctive features. Community/public health nursing is necessarily future-oriented; designing and implementing a healthy community agenda *now* will build its capacity to manage what may occur in 5, 10, or even 20 years.

Things happen more slowly in community/public health nursing. Compared with direct patient care, in which laboratory tests can be performed, reported, and acted upon in a matter of minutes, it often takes months, years, or decades to detect changes and trends in the health status of a community. An education program for teenage parents, for example, may not demonstrate a community-wide improvement in early-school performance of their children until at least 3 to 5 years after the program has been conceived and initiated. On the other hand, effectively designed community programs, such as those regarding community preparedness, may quickly address and evaluate the emergency management of the aftereffects of a community disaster. In public health practice, assessment, planning, intervention, and evaluation are ongoing, routine activities required to trace patterns of health, illness, and socio-demographic change in a community. The 5- and 10-year plans, revised annually through ongoing assessment, guide and organize the daily, weekly, and monthly activities of community health practice.

Suggested Activity

Compare and contrast the public health management of a rising incidence of environmentally associated neoplastic disease with the clinical management of the disease. Are public health management efforts effective and comprehensive? Why or why not?

The future and long-range orientation of community health practice poses some interesting dilemmas, because the real measure of effectiveness is not how well problems are handled as they occur but how successfully health is promoted and problems are averted. It is difficult to evaluate the effectiveness of community/public health nursing, because it often is measured by events that, if correctly addressed, will not happen. In addition, it is not always easy to engage community enthusiasm for results that may not occur for several months or even years.

On the other hand, when interventions to promote health and prevent disease are successfully in place, the magnitude of the results in terms of the hundreds, thousands, and even millions of people affected by public health interventions is thrilling and deeply gratifying for those fascinated by the opportunity to build sustainable communities, reshape healthcare, and ameliorate large-scale health problems. Immunizations, for example, are well recognized as the means for having greatly reduced morbidity and mortality from many infectious diseases. Polio, to name but one disease, has been nearly eradicated because of successful global public health efforts.

Suggested Activity

A local community has a growing population of non-English speaking migrants with complex but unmet health needs. What are examples of cultural capital that could be leveraged to facilitate the provision of culturally informed, accessible, and affordable health services?

By monitoring changes in the ethnic structure of the community's culture, we will be able to predict, for example, the following:

- In the next 5 years, the number of children under age 10 will increase dramatically.

- Many of those children will come from families in which English is a second language.

- A substantial proportion of those children will be in need of day care while their mothers are in the labor force.

- Much of the care for children with health problems will be carried out by teachers and school nurses.

- Neighborhoods with the greatest influx of children may have safety and health hazards that will affect child welfare and development.

This awareness of trends and the dynamic cultural matrix of the community is essential to anticipate, assess, plan, and prepare for emerging health issues, prevent health problems, promote health, and, critically important, build the cultural capacity to do so.

A Different Skill Set for Creating Health

Personal health services include a well-known range of nursing procedures that are the stock and trade of the clinician. Counseling a parent, changing a dressing, putting a patient through range-of-motion exercises, irrigating a catheter, and teaching a family member how to administer insulin are common procedures in the provision of direct patient care. Community/public health nursing intervention strategies, on the other hand, include public speaking, journalistic writing, social marketing, record keeping, statistical analyses, program development and evaluation, coalition building and political action, and policy formulation as the tasks performed by nurses to advocate for the health of a community. Interventions take place at the system level and might include promoting legislation to mandate exercise in school, being interviewed on a Spanish-language radio program, writing a guest column in the newspaper on how to select a nursing home, using social media (such as Twitter and Facebook) to promote health, using faith community newsletters to educate for better mental health services, mobilizing support for the cleanup of toxic waste, or analyzing data on sexually transmitted infections (STIs) as a means to secure support for sex education.

For example, several objectives in *Healthy People 2010* and in *Healthy People 2020* focus on the reduction of asthma, which is one of the top 10 reasons for emergency-department visits by children in the United States. In 2009, Bloom, Cohen, and Freeman reported that 23 million people in the United States had asthma, generating annual healthcare expenditures of $20.7 billion (National Heart, Lung, and Blood Institute, 2011). This number had increased to 25.5 million as of 2012 (Centers for Disease Control and Prevention, 2012). Although the number of deaths from asthma has decreased since the mid-1990s, the prevalence of asthma has continued to increase since 1980, particularly in low-income and minority populations, including women and children, African Americans, Puerto Ricans, and employees with workplace exposure. The care plan for a patient with asthma is likely to include breathing and relaxation exercises, inhalation therapy, one-to-one teaching, family counseling, and an emergency action plan. In contrast, the care plan for a community in which asthma is prevalent is likely to include identification of at-risk populations, implementation of screening programs, use of media resources for health education, smoking-cessation programs in schools and workplaces, public policy regulating air-pollution levels and smoke-free environments, and organization of community-action groups to lobby for better control of industrial wastes.

Similar Intervention, Different Application

Clinicians and community/public health nurses may use similar interventions, such as education, but apply them differently. For example, perioperative nurses provide individualized postsurgical instructions so the patient is informed of what to expect, what to do, where to go, and whom to ask for help in the event of an emergency. This education relieves anxiety, encourages rehabilitation, prevents complications, hastens recovery, and engages the patient in a therapeutic plan of care. Community/public health nurses, accountable for community-wide disaster preparedness, also use education as an intervention to ensure that residents and groups are aware of the disaster plan. To do this, they identify and deploy cultural capital, such as schools, radio and television stations, the chamber of commerce, and local grocery stores, in planning and disseminating the plan, establishing periodic disaster drills, enlisting and educating volunteers, publishing a website, and working with local merchants to stock a "disaster pack" of food, water, batteries, candles, and other necessities. With awareness of the community needs, these health-promotion and disease-prevention interventions are delivered in a culturally informed, literacy-appropriate, and evidence-based context.

STEPPING OUT OF HEALTHCARE: NEW PARTNERS IN PRACTICE

An important responsibility of clinicians is to work interprofessionally with other providers, such as the social worker, radiologist, physical therapist, physician, and lab technician, to increase efficiency and reduce the potential for error in patient care. In community health practice, partners from the fields of civic society, education, law enforcement, transportation, social services, and housing join public health in identifying, integrating, and deploying resources from every dimension of the community to promote the health of the public. These efforts might include bringing religious leaders of different denominations together with major industries to develop child-health and day care programs for working parents.

Similarly, legislators, industrial leaders, and emission experts could be convened to create policies that will improve the air quality of communities. Community/public health nurses collaborate with community partners from local organizations, media resources, and influential community leaders to create healthy communities. For example, the Federal Interagency Workgroup (FIW), which led the *Healthy People 2020* initiative, included not only the U.S. Department of Health & Human Services but also seven other federal agencies representing agriculture, education, housing and urban development, justice, interior, veterans' affairs, and the environment. This same model of community partnership happens at the local community level as well as on the national level.

COMMUNITY EVALUATION

In clinical practice, we evaluate our care to determine how successful we were in achieving the outcomes established by the client and the provider team. This could include recovering from an illness, becoming alcohol-free, reducing the number of emergency-department visits for a child with asthma, having an uncomplicated birth experience, or having a peaceful and meaningful death. Efficiency and cost enter the evaluation process in determining whether the same outcomes can be achieved at less cost or whether better outcomes can be achieved at the same cost. In community practice, the desired outcome is the extent to which cultural capital is used to achieve a healthier community—a place that is safer, cleaner, and more tolerant—where people live longer, more productive, and happier lives, and where health equity is being achieved. It is a dynamic process with ongoing evaluation interwoven with assessment and planning.

THE NURSE COMMUNITY PRESENCE: BUILDING RELATIONSHIPS

Community/public health nursing intervention is fundamentally a relationship-building exercise. Trusted alliances with community members and groups are essential for building community capacity and translating resources into a healthy community agenda. The process of engagement includes an openness to and integration of the diverse perspectives of community members.

VISIBILITY AND ROLE MODELING

The comparisons presented thus far suggest compelling differences in the nurse-client relationship in community/public health nursing practice. Unlike clinical practice, in which nurses see a relatively select category of patients (usually under very private circumstances), community/public health nurses develop ongoing, sustainable relationships and work with the whole population in everyday community life. It is important for community/public health nurses to be highly visible, taking part in community events and making themselves known to all sectors of the community and their leaders as credible resources who are invested in the care and well-being of the community. Through their reputation and relationships, they cultivate support for public health programs and policy reform.

Although all nurses, consciously or unconsciously, are role models for their clients, role modeling is particularly important for community/public health nurses. Constantly under the scrutiny of community residents, community nurses exemplify, in appearance and behavior, the expectations they set for community residents. How can community/public nurses launch a campaign to eliminate cigarette smoking in all public places if they are smokers themselves? How do community/public health nurses convince high-school administrators to initiate nutrition-education programs if they are overweight and have poor dietary habits? And how do community/public health nurses encourage citizens to vote and engage in public service unless they themselves are active participants in community public life?

CONFIDENTIALITY, UNIVERSALITY, AND TRUST

There is also the critical matter of confidentiality. Therapeutic relationships, grounded in trust and mutual respect, are essential for effective intervention in every nursing situation, whether in clinical or in public practice. It is, however, more complicated in community intervention, where the focus of practice is an entire community of people—some of whom may be at odds with one another or, at the very least, curious and cautious about one another. The betrayal of confidence with just one resident or community organization can generate a community-wide lack of trust and easily compromise acceptance and effectiveness of both the community/public health nurse and associated programs and activities. Maintaining confidentiality, abstaining from judgment, facilitating openness to diverse perspectives of community members, and developing an informed understanding of the culture of the community are essential skills for the practice of community/ public health nursing.

Unlike individual clients, communities are composed of many individuals and diverse groups who may have competing problems and conflicting goals and priorities. To be a potent force in achieving the public's health requires setting aside personal or group loyalties and working for the benefit of the community as a whole. Desired outcomes are achieved through coordination and articulation of community constituents and through win-win strategies. To do this, we must know the various groups and factions of the community, all of which must have—and know that they have—equal access to and the consideration of their community/public health nurse.

COMMUNITY/PUBLIC HEALTH NURSING VALUES

Chapter 1 concluded with three premises that form the moral construct of public health nursing: Health is a basic human right of all persons, healthy places are the starting point for healthy people, and community/public health nurses are accountable for system-level action to build community capacity and ensure social justice for health and healthcare. The statement that "health is a basic human right of all persons" is the core value that guides every component of community/ public health. This includes a practice that is culturally informed, purposefully engages all citizen groups, builds on the strengths of these sectors, and is evaluated based on health equity and social justice.

But the fact that communities are composed of groups with conflicting goals and competing values creates unique ethical issues in public health practice. Indeed, one of the most distinguishing features of community/public health nursing is its value orientation, in which the *common good* takes precedence over the good of the individual (ANA, 2007). The community/public health nurse who provides personal health services and community-level intervention often is caught in a web of competing values. This tension between the individual and society in ensuring the public's health has always existed. Ruth Freeman, a founding leader in community/public health nursing education in the United States, addressed this explicitly in 1963:

> The selection of those to be served … must rest on the compara-
> tive impact on community health rather than solely on the needs
> of the individual or family being served…. The community health
> nurse cannot elect to care for a small number of people intensely
> while ignoring the needs of many others. She [*sic*] must be con-
> cerned with the community as a whole. (p. 35)

This passage leaves no room for doubt: Grounded in utilitarian ethics, when there is conflict between individual goals and community goals, community goals must prevail. Such conflicts typically arise when there is competition for limited health resources.

Consider a community in which a small number of individuals could benefit from the presence of sophisticated cardiac technology in a local hospital. The families of these individuals and their cardiologists may present a strong case for having these procedures available locally. On the other hand, the community may achieve more enduring, less costly, and better outcomes if limited resources were directed toward the *prevention* of cardiac disease, such as a community-based recreation facility and a cardiac health education program to instruct all families in the community on the principles of good cardiac health.

There are times when community/public health nurses may have to select among competing goals, all of which are for the good of the whole. Communities are complex aggregates, and although some values are shared among all residents, groups within the community may disagree about particular issues and events. Therefore, there are bound to be occasions of conflict not only between individual- and community-level objectives but also among different factions within communities.

With these opposing demands, how does one define the common good? The good of the whole community does not necessarily mean the desires of the majority. Imagine, for example, a community in which a particular industry, which happens to be the largest employer of community residents, is engaged in a conflict with the health department and concerned citizens regarding its dangerous waste-disposal practices. If compliance with waste-disposal regulations has economic consequences for employees, such as reductions in workforce or decreased wages, it is likely that the offending industry will have many supporters in the conflict while the health department will have only a few, despite the more enduring value of its position for the health of the community. Caring for the health of the public requires not only a shift in the practice paradigm but also a shift in the values that influence priority setting and decision-making when faced with the inevitable conflict between individual and public health and among special-interest stakeholders within communities. The ways in which community/public health nursing resources (time, expertise, experience, and influence) are deployed must reflect the whole community now and in the future.

3

LEARNING THE CULTURE AND HEALTH OF COMMUNITIES

A comprehensive understanding of the community—its health and its culture—is the foundation for building community capacity. Assessment, the first of the three core public health functions, is a prerequisite to assurance and policy. This chapter describes how to gather information about the culture and the health of a whole community using *ethnography* and *epidemiology*, two strategies for collecting, organizing, and analyzing information that inform community/public health practice in different but complementary ways.

CHAPTER 3 OBJECTIVES

- Describe how ethnography and epidemiology inform the assessment of the culture and health of a community.

- Know the strategies and techniques for collecting, organizing, and analyzing information about the community and its health.

- Identify the types and sources of information about the community.

LEARNING ABOUT THE COMMUNITY'S CULTURE AND HEALTH

Community/public health nurses who have worked with the same community for a long time have institutional memories about generations of residents, the environment, politics, the economy, and healthcare. Having internalized all of this cultural information, their decisions tend to be highly effective but generally grounded in experience rather than evidence. To be useful for community decision-makers, we need a documented and comprehensive assessment of the community, its culture, and its health. Although community/public health nurses are responsible for ongoing community data collection and management, they are not researchers. Their goal is not to develop or test new knowledge but rather to assemble a community inventory of its problems *and* its cultural capital. A culturally informed community health assessment will reveal appropriate and effective ways to intervene and promote the health of the community.

A *community culture assessment* is the routine and systematic collection, management, analysis, and organization of information required for culturally informed planning and action. In clinical practice, patient interventions ordinarily are preceded by an assessment and followed by an evaluation. In public health, however, the collection and management of community data are ongoing activities required to ensure the accessibility of accurate information when needed. Ethical, cost-effective, and sustainable community health services necessitate an ongoing inventory of various aspects of life in the community for more beneficial community planning.

Conducting an assessment of the community's culture also provides an important opportunity to become acquainted with community residents and build trusting relationships. Although it may be impossible to interact directly with every member of the community, it is essential to establish an acquaintance and a presence with all sectors of the community. This includes informal groups, such as the "regulars" at the local coffee shop, members of the Red Hat society, or a mothers' morning playgroup at the recreation center. It also includes community leaders from business, education, law enforcement, and religious institutions as well as representatives of particular ethnic constituencies. Building relationships with community residents and collecting accurate and useful information are mutually reinforcing activities.

INFORMING PUBLIC HEALTH PRACTICE THROUGH ETHNOGRAPHY

Ethnographic inquiry yields a broad understanding of the sociocultural factors that affect health and illness and how they are related. It requires long-term immersion in and observation of community life to capture the perspective of the local people. The goal of ethnography in public health practice is to reveal the factors that collectively influence the community's health and the health of its individual citizens. Using the whole community as the unit of analysis, ethnographic descriptions and comparisons explore such questions as which local factors distinguish neighborhoods with a high rate of childhood asthma from those with a low rate? How is childhood asthma linked to factors of local life? Where and when are highest number of asthma emergencies recorded? Which children are most likely to be affected? What are the dynamics between childhood asthma and social class or between asthma and social institutions, such as education and recreation? Ethnographic descriptions identify the dynamic cultural matrix in which illness is caused and health is produced.

As we learned in Chapter 1, ethnographic strategies also identify culture-specific solutions gleaned from the community's cultural capital. So how do we begin to acquire an understanding of our community's culture? Using ethnography (Bernard, 2011), our investigation begins with the big picture of the whole community as the *object* of intervention (for long-range community health planning) and the *context* of intervention (the *place* and *time* in which specific problems are addressed) (Arensberg, 1961; Drevdahl, 1999). Before we begin working on a particular health issue or problem—whether it is low-birth-weight infants, obesity, air pollution, disaster preparedness, or safety for older adults—we need to understand communities as constellations of *physical environment, population,* and *social organization,* in which we can explore specific public health problems.

If, for example, epidemiological studies indicate that obesity in preschool-age children in our community is increasing, we would want to find out which families in our community have this problem, where they live, and how they live. Are they distributed throughout the community, or are they concentrated in particular neighborhoods or income groups? How do the families of these children intersect with the larger community? Where do they work and recreate, and how do they procure and prepare food? What is different about these families from similar families in which preschool-age children are not obese? Perhaps most important, we would want to know what it is like to be a preschool-age child in this community: Who cares for them during the day and prepares their food? What and where do they eat? Where and with whom do they play? Were they breastfed or bottle-fed? Do they go to day care or to preschool programs? What amount and kind of physical activity do they get during the day? Gathering information about this population *in the context of its community* gives us a better understanding of the complexity and interconnectedness of the problem and the cultural capital needed to address it.

GATHERING COMMUNITY DATA

When we conduct a health assessment on an individual patient, we review a combination of laboratory data, patient reports, and provider observations. Similarly, community health assessments combine many kinds of objective and subjective data as well as quantitative and qualitative data, each of which contributes to a comprehensive understanding of the community and a basis for interpretation of health and illness. In community health practice, there are three main sources of community assessment data:

■ What we observe directly about the community

■ What is documented about the community in newspapers, radio and television, historical sources, census reports, vital records and bio-statistical reports, epidemiological surveys, and websites

■ What people tell us about the community

WHAT WE OBSERVE DIRECTLY

Before we begin the process of building relationships in our community, we can learn a great deal simply by touring the community and mapping its various components. Is there, for example, a "downtown" with businesses, residential areas, or suburbs that require owning an automobile? Are there topographical features that define the community physically and perhaps economically, such as rivers, mountains, or prairie? Or a built environment, such as super-highways, bridges, or boardwalks, that can separate and unite various components of the community? To have an understanding of the physical community, it is useful to have at least three maps:

- One that outlines the major topographical features of the community (e.g., mountain ranges, hills, rivers, lakes and ponds, and seashore)

- One that designates the regional position of the district/community in relation to urban centers and outlines the transportation system in and out of the community

- One that denotes settlement patterns, streets, highways, residential areas, and commercial areas

Use these maps to post observable products of physical culture, such as schools, parks, theaters, docks, public administration buildings, police precincts, businesses, hospitals, museums, temples, churches, mosques, and residential dwellings—houses, apartment buildings, and neighborhood designations. This is also an opportunity to observe differences of prosperity within the community. Posting the vulnerable aspects of the community on these maps (e.g., tracts of poor housing, congested streets, personal-injury crimes, environmental hazard areas, polluted water, and so on) as you walk through the community begins to create a visual representation of the environmental and social health of the community.

Suggested Activity

Use Internet mapping tools, such as http://earth.google.com, as well as paper and pencil to sketch out the landmarks as you drive and walk around the community.

The way in which residents organize and use time is another observable aspect of culture and equally as important as their use of space. Observing people as they come and go at different times of the day and week in different schedules and cycles of activities to work or school or recreation is revealing. Are there industrial plants in which three shifts of employees are working, or does everyone leave the community in the morning and return every evening? Who are the people who remain there while others are at work? Which days of the week are reserved for worship? For schooling? For commercial activities? How do people get around the community—by private vehicles or by public transportation? Who is attending public events, celebrations, and holidays and religious festivals that provide excellent opportunities to see the community in action and the seasonal and annual rhythms of local culture? It is useful to record these aspects of community life on daily, weekly, and annual schedules and calendars. People use their communities 24 hours a day, 7 days a week, and all seasons of the year. Ethnographic observations of people in relation to time capture important issues of public health, such as traffic congestion, availability of emergency care, parental supervision of food consumption, seasonal environmental hazards, dangerous behavior associated with celebrations, school vacation injuries, and so forth.

Suggested Activity

Post community events and cycles on an annual calendar. Post patterns of community activities on weekly and monthly schedules.

Attending routine community events, such as public hearings, religious services, and parent-teacher association meetings, and visiting shopping centers, school playgrounds, train stations, and movie theaters reveal the culture of local life and group-held values. The goal is to be as comprehensive as possible. The calendar/schedules and the various maps are working documents, always being revised and updated. The most useful calendars and maps are likely to look cluttered and even chaotic as more data are added. They will, however, provide a highly useful visual inventory of the community's use of space and time over a year and its implications for public health.

A family-planning project designed to bring contraception education to rural Caribbean communities included a fully equipped van with an electric generator, a film projector, and a full assemblage of family-planning materials. Family-planning educators were selected, trained, and scheduled to visit several communities each week. The presentations were usually scheduled in the evening on a weeknight and were ordinarily filled to capacity. The attendees, however, were mostly older children and men—the women of childbearing age were home looking after their small children. Although it is certainly advantageous for all community residents to be exposed to the concept of family planning, the target population for whom the program was intended was not there. The program planners had neglected to take into consideration that in these rural communities, men are nighttime gatherers, while women are daytime gatherers. Had the program been held on Sunday at various churches in the community, in the marketplace on Saturday, or at rural clinics on a weekday, it is likely more women of childbearing age would have been reached.

A word about first observations of the communities we will be serving: Our initial impressions are not always accurate and often change dramatically once we get to know our places and people. Peace Corps workers reported being overwhelmed by the crowded streets, poorly clothed people, disrepair of the homes, and freely wandering goats and pigs on first entering some of the communities to which they were assigned. After being in their respective locations for several weeks, however, and exposed to other communities, they often reclassified their communities from "impoverished" to "working class." They learned that best clothes were reserved for religious days, houses were modest but not in dangerous disrepair, and while toilets were outside, they were clean and serviceable. The families in these communities had access to resources, including livestock; were sending their children to school; and were making strides toward social and economic improvement in a complex environment.

Regardless of which communities we enter as public health professionals, impressions are subject to observer bias or prejudgment and will change as we come to know more about the communities and their cultures. It is important, nonetheless, to record first observations and occasionally return to them. In the process of becoming familiar with a community, one begins to take some of its characteristics for granted. Our first impressions help us understand the reactions of newcomers and retain objectivity about the community to which we already have become accustomed.

WHAT IS DOCUMENTED ABOUT THE COMMUNITY

Documents are one of the best ways to back up your observations with facts. Good starting points include the size of the community's population and its characteristics in terms of age, sex, education, income, religious affiliation, and language groups. The numbers and types of homes, businesses, religious denominations, schools, hospitals, medical practices, and so forth are often documented in official records, as are the number of marriages, divorces, home purchases, bankruptcy filings, arrests, deaths, births, graduations, and car sales. All of these data provide a rich picture of human activity in a particular township, village, or city.

Many communities—especially those that are geo-political units—have a web page. Although such web pages ordinarily portray the town, city, or county in the best possible light, they are still useful for acquiring a preliminary picture of self-identified community strengths and are a good starting point for your ethnographic inquiry. Newspapers provide an excellent introduction to the community's culture, including local advertisement-based papers available in grocery stores and real-estate offices. If the community does not have a newspaper of its own, the closest local newspaper will reveal the way in which the community is perceived regionally. *Yellow Pages* of the telephone directory, now online, list hospitals, churches, recreational facilities, schools, day care centers, physicians, lawyers, businesses, and other services for residents that are useful in an inventory of community resources and cultural capital.

There are many other formal centers of community information, including the local library, the chamber of commerce, government offices, department of education, police and fire departments, and parks and recreation offices. City- or county-planning commissions, if they exist, are particularly valuable. A benefit of personally visiting local organizations is the opportunity to meet the most knowledgeable members of the community, inform them of the community health assessment, and obtain the most up-to-date information sources. A good source of socio-demographic data can be obtained from the most recent census (United States Census Bureau, 2016). Finally, geo-politically defined communities and their constituent institutions (schools, libraries, and civic organizations) produce annual reports and may have several reports dating back decades or even centuries that will give you a sense of the history of a community that will help you understand its contemporary culture.

A problem in using documents prepared by various community public services is that they often are in units that are not coterminous with each other or with your designated community. Information pertaining to children may have been compiled by school districts, data on communicable disease may have been compiled according to health districts, and data on public sanitation and safety may have been compiled according to fire and water districts or police districts. This variance is particularly true in more complex urban environments, where public institutions and offices have sliced the pies of state, county, or city in different ways. Not only are these various districts not coterminous: They may cut across census tracks as well as community boundaries. The use of these data will require some exercise in judgment and an acknowledgment that some data are better than no data. Finally, formal and informal documentation can be copied and/or saved and added to the maps and calendars in the community health field notes, which we discuss later in the chapter. Newspaper clippings, real-estate ads, and formal census documents all contribute information to a comprehensive assessment of community culture.

WHAT PEOPLE TELL US ABOUT THE COMMUNITY

Meeting and talking with people who reside in or are familiar with the community are also important sources of cultural information. Ethnographers refer to such persons as "informants" in the sense that they *inform* us about the world they know or in which they live. Each person's perspective will reflect his or her particular position in the community, including, for example, length of residence, occupation, neighborhood, age, sex, and socioeconomic status. We should not be surprised, therefore, when different members of the community give very different—even conflicting—reports about the same community issue or event. One person may claim her neighborhood is changing for the worse, while another may describe it as revitalized and an exciting place to live.

The greater the number and variety of community residents you meet and talk with, the more complete the picture of the community's culture. Unlike clinical practice, most of the persons with whom the community/public health nurse interacts—for example, public officials, religion leaders, teachers, librarians, politicians, merchants, industrialists, restaurant owners, bartenders, real-estate brokers, bankers, journalists, or police officers—are *not* in healthcare and thus have a different vision of the community. Each of these persons will view the community through a different lens, and each is equally valid. Their collective narrative about the community—its culture, its strengths, and its opportunities—provides a deeper and broader understanding of culture.

In ethnographic inquiry, subjective reports from community members are highly useful if the names and positions of the individuals are recorded along with what they say. Capturing the diversity of opinions and sources of conflict provides great insight into the micropolitics of local life and culture, and knowing the status and role of the particular informant helps us interpret what is really going on, especially when recording the actual words. Compare, for example, the following excerpts taken from the field notes of two students recording the same event:

> At the Centerville Town Meeting, Mr. Johnson, principal of Centerville High School, stated that he would not support Representative Snyder in the next election, because she opposed the introduction of sex education in the public school system.

> Educators from Centerville H.S. engaged in a lively discussion about sex education and local politics.

In the first statement, the relationships linking education, politics, and sex education are clear, not just from the perspective of any community resident but also from one who holds a pivotal position and works in all three arenas. This more specific statement helps us understand current political issues, draw inferences about local sexual mores, and know who would or would not support programs that address the issue of adolescent sexuality. In conducting a community ethnography, it is necessary to know not only what was said or written but who said or wrote it.

One last word about using conversational data: The reliability of what people tell us must always be evaluated. People have various reasons for sharing different pieces of information, and some people are going to be more credible than others. The role of the community/public health nurse engaged in conversation is always to listen and never to repeat. For almost every piece of information that someone is willing, perhaps eager, to share, it is always good to decide, "Why is this person giving me this information?" and "Why *now*?" This approach is not cynical—it just recognizes how human communities work.

WHAT IS THE BEST SOURCE OF DATA FOR UNDERSTANDING COMMUNITY CULTURE?

The relative value of some sources of information over others is simply a function of their usefulness in addressing the question being asked. For example, if the public health concern being addressed is the nutritional status of schoolchildren, there are several approaches to understanding the problem:

- We could ask children to complete a questionnaire on their 24-hour nutritional intake.

- We could review the school menus over the past 3 months and evaluate the nutritional content of the meals.

- We could rely on direct observations of eating behavior and food consumption by schoolchildren during mealtimes.

Each of these sources of information has advantages and disadvantages. In the 24-hour nutritional intake, the children may consciously or unconsciously report wholesome-food consumption and neglect to mention the candy bar or potato chips purchased from a vending machine. School menus provide reliable information on what was served, but not on what was actually eaten. Direct observations, in this case, are probably the most revealing source of information but are very expensive to collect, because you cannot observe all the children at the same time. The most complete and easily obtained picture of the problem is derived from a combination of the three sources of information.

For some kinds of public health issues, direct observations may not be the best source of information. For example, if we were formulating a 5-year plan for the provision of prenatal services in a specific community, observations and interviews with childbearing women in prenatal clinics may be much less useful than census reports and data on migration patterns, economic changes, and birth and infant statistics over the past decade. Different sources of data also permit the examination of values and behaviors and the discrepancies that often exist between what people say and what people do. For example, community members may report that they value good health and believe cigarette smoking is bad—yet continue to smoke. Teachers may instruct children in the principles of good nutrition in the classroom but not raise objections to the installation of a candy vending machine in the school cafeteria to increase school revenues. Identifying discrepancies and conflicts between what people say and what people do is critical to designing community health action plans that work. They reveal the cultural realities and the conflicted nature of human social existence.

Again, no matter which sources of data are included for the community assessment, it is always more helpful to report specific behavior and events than general impressions. In clinical practice, the information recorded in the patient's chart is expected to be exactly what is observed and heard. The same expectation applies to public health. Compare these two examples:

Last year, there were 22 incidents of assault and robbery in which the victim was 75 years or older, in comparison with 5 years earlier, when there were none.

Victimization of elders is a growing problem in this community.

Specific information citing the growing incidence of crimes against older adult citizens helps bolster the argument for securing resources for older citizens, such as low-cost transit service or increased police surveillance. In addition to recording community observations and conversation, it is important to critically review the information in documents. Every type of information has inherent strengths, biases, and limitations that are important to acknowledge when designing a culturally informed community health assessment. Similar to the information that comes from what people tell us, documented and published information also reflects the perspective of the people and organizations who wrote and published them and the purposes for which they were to be used. Local newspapers, for example, necessarily reflect the political and philosophical biases of the editors. Material assembled by the chamber of commerce attempts to cast the community in a positive light to attract businesses. Information collected by the health department, on the other hand, may be oriented more to community health concerns.

COMMUNITY HEALTH FIELD NOTES

Ethnographic data are recorded in field notes, which are typed up routinely and retained in a fieldwork notebook. They reflect ongoing observations of and interactions with the community: the physical environment, population, and social organization. For community/public health nurses, community health field notebooks provide a comprehensive narrative about their clients—the community—over time, to which they can refer as the need arises. There are several equally useful formats for community health field notes, but every format should include:

- The date, time, and name of the event being recorded;

- A description of the event (place, people, and activities);

- A place for indexing (the kind of event—politics, health, education, or any others that apply) so that you can organize your notes topically for specific initiatives;

- Personal comments (if cogent) and follow-up (if any); and

- The date on which the notes were recorded (if different from the date on which the event occurred).

Not unlike clinical nursing—where you document your assessment, plan, care, and evaluation prior to leaving the clinic or hospital setting—it is important to document your community information on the same day it is collected. The memory loss in just 1 day is exponential and compromises the cultural information you will want to share with the rest of the team. Organizing this information allows you to access all the cultural information about a specific health initiative (e.g., school safety, senior health, prenatal care). It will guide the identification and analysis of community cultural capital and culturally informed programming and evaluation. The following example of community field notes may be helpful:

Time	Date and Event: May 1, 2015	Index	Personal Comments	Follow-Up
9:30 am	**Meeting with school principal, Mrs. Hazard, to discuss healthy lunches program.** 3 years in role, came from neighboring community, teaching social studies for 8 years, master's in school admin	Child Nutrition Schools	Had trouble making this appointment. Canceled three times.	Meet with school board to get big picture.

	Described the pressure from school board chair to adhere to budget. He regards healthy lunches as a "luxury."	Principal	She was cordial but guarded.	Discuss possible role of nursing students to meet needs of kids with chronic illness with university faculty.
	She does not want to install unhealthy vending machines. She got along very well with the previous board chair, "whose focus was the welfare of the children." The current board chair "not so much." Concerned more about reducing taxes.	School Board School Nurses	I felt she was appealing to me to meet with board chair and try to convince him. Meeting ended well. Agreed to follow up in a couple weeks with ideas on how nursing school could serve children with chronic illness: Student practice experience? Faculty practice?	
	She listed competing needs— specifically computers, Internet, library updates, staff person to manage increasing number of children with chronic illnesses on medications and procedures.			
	Didn't have a strategic plan from which to budget.			
11:00 am	Meeting ended		Excellent meeting. Worth waiting for.	Schedule revisit in 3 months.

INFORMING COMMUNITY/PUBLIC HEALTH PRACTICE THROUGH EPIDEMIOLOGY AND BIO-STATISTICS

The primary goal of epidemiology is to determine the causes and risk factors of disease and other health problems by identifying and analyzing their distribution among *designated populations*. Statistics uses numbers to summarize information or data that are collected in the community. Traditionally, the health of communities was measured almost exclusively by the presence or absence of disease in its population—especially acute, infectious disease. Epidemiology, originally the study of epidemics, has now expanded to include chronic illness and other health and social problems, such as crime rates, automobile injuries, substandard housing, high-school graduation rates, and health disparities. One research area of epidemiology is to identify the risk factors (e.g., age, ethnicity, tobacco use, obesity, sex) associated with prevailing public health problems. Based on the outcomes, screening programs are implemented for early detection of these risk factors and early community intervention.

Epidemiology also identifies populations known as high-risk groups—that is, groups that are especially vulnerable to specific illnesses. Risk groups can be associated with many kinds of factors, such as biological (breast cancer in women), ethnic (diabetes in some Native American groups), socioeconomic (high rates of asthma in children of families living below the poverty level), and occupational (chemical exposure in the workplace). Epidemiological data are usually presented using bio-statistics. Before we discuss the contribution of epidemiology to a community health assessment, a brief summary of some of the basic bio-statistical measures of population health is useful.

BIO-STATISTICAL MEASURES OF POPULATION HEALTH

Birth, death (mortality), and illness (morbidity) statistics ordinarily are expressed as *rates* rather than absolute numbers, because rates enable comparison of the experience of populations with one another as well as across timeframes. Each rate is computed by dividing the number of events in question—for example, death by suicide—occurring during a specific time period by the population at risk for the event during the same time period. The phrase "population at risk" means all those persons who have the potential to experience the health problem in question. For example, because women do not have the potential to contract testicular cancer, they would not be counted among the population at risk for morbidity or mortality for that disease. But because all members of a population have the potential for dying, death rates are calculated using the entire population as the denominator.

CALCULATING RATES

$$\text{RATE} = \frac{\text{The number of specified events during a particular time period}}{\text{The population at risk for the event at midpoint during the time period}} \times 1,000, 10,000, 100,000$$

The numerator and denominator used to calculate rates must reflect the same population in the same time period, with the numerator being included in the denominator. The number in the denominator is computed by using the population at the midpoint of the specified time period.

Rates are expressed as multiples of 100, 1,000, 10,000, or 100,000. The choice of multiplicative factor depends on the size of the population and the frequency with which the event occurs. The rates should be expressed in a figure that is not so small that it must be expressed in a fraction or so large that it is awkward or unwieldy. For example, the mortality rate of AIDS in the early years of the epidemic in the United States was given as a multiple of 1,000, because cases were few at that time. Currently, the rate is expressed per 100,000; this reflects the increase in diagnosed cases over the past 20 years. For example, to express the rate of AIDS for a specific city of 500,000 inhabitants in which there were five reported cases of AIDS, the morbidity rate would be .01 per 1,000, or 1 per 100,000. Although both calculations express the same information and thus could theoretically be used interchangeably, 1 per 100,000 is the least cumbersome and most broadly applied. Convention also tends to dictate the multiplicative factor. Infant mortality rates, for example, are commonly expressed using 1,000 as the multiplicative factor, while maternal mortality rates, reflecting a less-frequent event, are usually expressed using 10,000. In any case, the multiplicative factor should always be mentioned when reporting the rate.

By looking at the rate rather than the absolute number of occurrences, groups of different sizes may be compared to determine the relative severity of the problem in any population. For most purposes, raw numbers are not useful in a community health assessment, because they do not lend themselves to comparison with other communities and populations, and thus their significance is obscured. In other words, it is impossible to know whether the number of cases is low or high relative to other communities or whether it represents a major departure from previous numbers for that community.

Crude Rates

Crude rates, which have not been adjusted to account for age or other factors, may yield unjustifiable conclusions. For example, it would be misguided to compare the crude death rate in a retirement community with that of a community in which elders represent only 5% of the population.

$$\text{CRUDE DEATH RATE} = \frac{\text{The number of deaths}}{\text{Total population}} \times 100,000$$

To make such a comparison, it would be necessary to adjust for the age factor to produce a standardized rate, called an age-adjusted rate. An age-adjusted rate is calculated by adjusting (or weighting) the crude rate by the proportion of persons in the age group in a population. Because age is the single best predictor of overall mortality and morbidity, the age adjustment of mortality and morbidity rates is crucial for evaluative purposes (Hebel & McCarter, 2006). Many different kinds of rates can be used to describe the health status of a population—for example, age-specific rates (the rate of teenage death), sex-specific rates (the rate of alcoholism among females), or any other possible subgrouping of a larger population. The denominator in these instances is only the number of people in the specified subgroup.

An understanding of statistical rates and how they are calculated is important to assessing the health of a population. In clinical nursing, clients' vital signs provide gross but immediate and important indications of their well-being. In population assessment, the vital signs are health-status indicators that include not only mortality and morbidity rates but also many of the statistics presented in Chapter 5,

"Discovering the Culture of Your Community," and Chapter 6, "Determining the Health of Your Community." For example, poverty rates, unemployment rates, and the percentage of the population on public assistance all help predict the kinds and numbers of health problems in any given population. The Centers for Disease Control and Prevention (CDC) has recommended a standard set of health-status indicators to be used by each state (http://wwwn.cdc.gov/communityhealth). It is critical for community/public health providers to know whether their states have developed this kind of instrument and how to access it.

Selecting the health-status indicators that will provide the most relevant information about the health of a community depends largely on the community and the concerns of its residents. For example, using maternal-child health statistics to measure the well-being of a retirement community would not be very useful, nor would it be helpful to rely as heavily on chronic disease rates to evaluate the health status of a developing country that is more affected by infectious diseases.

Mortality Rates

Mortality rates measure the number and categories of deaths. Whereas crude death rates are based on the entire population, specific mortality rates relate to the number of deaths in various categories, such as a particular subgroup of the population (e.g., children, an ethnic group) or deaths from specified causes (e.g., accidents, cancer). It is not unusual for the top three causes of death in a particular community to be consistent with national statistics. In most states, death rates are highest for cardiovascular disease, cancer, and stroke. The most local variation is likely to occur in the remaining mortality rates; they provide the most significant information regarding the health status of a particular community.

$$\text{CAUSE SPECIFIC DEATH RATE} = \frac{\text{Total number of deaths from a specified cause}}{\text{Total population}} \times 1{,}000,\ 10{,}000,\ 100{,}000$$

Suggested Activity

List the age-adjusted rates for the five leading causes of death in your community.

- How do these rates compare with the rates for the previous 5 and 10 years?
- How do these rates compare with state and national rates?
- What trends and differences are present, and how can they be explained?

Morbidity Rates

Unlike mortality rates, which are concerned with the numbers and kinds of deaths in a population, *morbidity rates* are concerned with the occurrence of various diseases or health problems in a population. Thus, the number of people who die from cancer is reflected in the mortality rate, while the number of people who are diagnosed with cancer is expressed in the morbidity rate.

Morbidity rates are reported in terms of incidence and prevalence. *Incidence* refers to the number of newly reported cases that occur during a specified period of time. *Prevalence*, on the other hand, is more of a snapshot approach; it refers to the total number of cases (new and old) that exist in a specified period of time. If, for example, a total of 20 new cases of diabetes in a population of 10,000 were reported during 2004, the incidence rate for that year would be 20 per 10,000 (or 2 per 1,000). Because those 20 join the ranks of the 180 individuals already diagnosed with diabetes, swelling the total number to 200, the prevalence rate for diabetes in the district would be 200 per 10,000 (or 20 per 1,000).

Occasionally, one sees reference to an attack rate. This is a subcategory of the incidence rate and refers to a very limited period of time. For example, one might use the attack rate to measure the effects of an outbreak of salmonella poisoning or measles during a specific period.

Incidence and prevalence rates have different uses. Incidence rates are used for the following reasons:

- To determine etiology or causation

- To identify trends in disease occurrence

When the incidence rate rises, we suspect that a new etiological agent (or cause) is operative or that the etiological factors already known have increased in amount or virulence.

The prevalence rate, on the other hand, is used to plan for health services. It gives a current picture of the total number of people who are alive with the illness at a given point in time.

$$\text{INCIDENCE} = \frac{\text{Number of new cases of a disease or health problem occurring during a specified period of time}}{\text{Population at risk at midpoint in time period}} \times 1{,}000, 10{,}000, 100{,}000$$

$$\text{PREVALENCE} = \frac{\text{Total number of cases of a disease or health problem occurring during a specified time period}}{\text{Total population at midpoint in time period}} \times 1{,}000, 10{,}000, 100{,}000$$

An increase in the prevalence rate can reflect an increase in incidence plus duration—that is, there are more cases than usual and/or more successful treatment outcomes that result in more people with the illness surviving for longer periods of time. Thus, decreases in the prevalence rate may be due to death or to the discovery of curative treatments. New treatment methods alone do not influence the prevalence rate, unless they are successful in curing the illness.

From the size and composition of the population, it is possible to anticipate the amount and the content of health services needed now and in the future. Morbidity data address health problems even more directly and refine predictions of population health status. Both incidence and prevalence rates are important and useful, because they give very different kinds of information about the presence of illness in the community. Unfortunately, they often are difficult to obtain at the local level, because doing so requires surveying the population, which is very time-consuming and expensive. Usually, only incidence rates for reportable infectious diseases, such as AIDS, tuberculosis, sexually transmitted infections (STIs), and cancer, are available for local communities. In addition, when the total population of a community is very small, the health department often will not publish these rates for privacy reasons.

Suggested Activity

List the incidence and prevalence rates of the five leading causes of death in your community.

- How do they compare with the rates for the previous 5 and 10 years?
- How do they compare with state and national rates?
- What trends and differences are present, and how can they be explained?
- Which populations are disproportionately affected by infectious disease?

EPIDEMIOLOGICAL STUDIES OF POPULATION HEALTH

Monitoring the incidence rate is critical for identifying etiology and new causes (or causal agents). Because the resources for doing this often are not sufficient, epidemiological research strategies correlate suspected risk factors with the occurrence of disease when the population incidence rates are not available. These research approaches are known as *case-control (or retrospective) studies* and *cohort (or prospective) studies*.

CASE-CONTROL STUDIES

When disease prevalence is low in the population or there are limited funds with which to investigate, a case-control study, also referred to as a retrospective study, may be conducted. Some of the most commonly accepted risk factors have been implicated as a result of case-control studies, including smoking and lung cancer and family history and breast cancer.

Case-control studies can be carried out in a reasonably short period of time and are the most economical to conduct. They identify two groups of people—one with the disease and one without. These groups are further subdivided into those who have been exposed to the suspected etiological agent and those who have not. This comparison yields a statistic called an *odds ratio* (OR), which calculates the odds of having the disease when the suspected factor is present as opposed to absent.

Odds ratios are estimations of a statistic called the *relative risk* (RR), which can be calculated only when the true incidence rate of a disease is available. The higher the odds ratio or relative risk, the more likely the suspected etiologic factor is causally related to disease incidence. In the case of breast cancer, for example, historically, three factors consistently identified by case-control studies with an odds ratio of greater than 4 are (a) older age, (b) birth in a North American or northern European country, and (c) having a family history (mother and/or sister) of breast cancer (Cuzick, 2003). The latter two factors strongly suggest either a genetic or an environmental etiology; in fact, a gene for breast cancer has been isolated.

Impetus for exploring this genetic line of research was no doubt prompted by the strong association found in many case-control studies that linked breast cancer to family history and country of origin. Other well-publicized risk factors for breast cancer, such as multiparity, early age at menarche, late age at menopause, and alcohol consumption, have lower relative risk—between 1.1 and 2 (Cuzick, 2003).

Case-Control Study

Suppose 220 women with breast cancer are recruited for a study and are compared with 1,140 women who do not have the disease. The total group is further divided into those who have a sister or mother who has breast cancer (exposure present) and those who do not (exposure absent). Typically, a case-control study is depicted as a 2-by-2 table.

Disease

		Present	Absent	Totals
	Present	100(a)	150(b)	250
Exposure				
	Absent	120(c)	990(d)	1,100

*The equation for establishing an odds ratio is as follows:

$$OR = \frac{ad}{bc}$$

$$OR = \frac{99,000}{18,000} = 5.5$$

Thus, the odds of someone with a mother or sister with breast cancer being diagnosed with the same disease in this sample are 5.5 times greater than for someone without a similar family history.

COHORT STUDIES

When sufficient evidence exists to suggest a link between a factor and a disease, a cohort study may be proposed. This type of study, also referred to as longitudinal, examines the disease experience of a cohort of people over time. Cohort studies can be historical, in which case the records of large groups of people exposed to a certain risk (for example, workers in an asbestos manufacturing plant) are examined for past levels of exposure and disease occurrence. They also can be prospective, in which case a total population or representative sample is followed over time, and morbidity and mortality rates are related to study variables.

Much of what is known about risk factors for coronary heart disease comes from an ongoing prospective study begun in Framingham, Massachusetts, in 1949 (https://www.framinghamheartstudy.org). Cohort studies of this type are very useful but often prohibitively expensive. Using the cohort design, a relative risk can be calculated by dividing the incidence rate of a disease among those exposed by the incidence rate among those not exposed. Thus, relative risk measures the strength of the association between a factor and an outcome (Hebel & McCarter, 2006). Again, the higher the odds ratio or relative risk, the more likely the factor being studied is causal or etiological.

Causal relationships are demonstrated even more strongly by calculating the difference in disease occurrence in groups exposed to the factor to different degrees—for example, comparing the odds ratios or relative risks from case-control or cohort studies for lung cancer in those who smoked one, two, and three packs of cigarettes a day. If greater exposure results in a higher odds ratio or relative risk, a dose-response relationship is established, with causality more likely. In fact, this is exactly how the now widely accepted causal relationship between smoking and lung cancer was established.

Cohort Study

A group of nurses is followed for 40 years, from first licensure until the present, and the occurrence of lung cancer is recorded. A total of 40,000 nurses are enrolled in the study, and they are divided into smokers and nonsmokers.

Disease

	Lung Cancer	No Lung Cancer	Total
Smokers	1,400(a)	14,600(b)	16,000
Risk Factor			
Nonsmokers	200(c)	23,800(d)	24,000

The equation for calculating the relative risk is as follows:

$$\text{Relative Risk} = \frac{\text{incidence rate among exposed}}{\text{incidence rate among nonexposed}}$$

Thus, in this case, the equation reads as follows:

$$RR = \frac{a/(a+b)}{c/(c+d)} = \frac{1,400/16,000}{200/24,000} = 10.5$$

In this sample, it can be concluded that the probability of developing lung cancer is 10.5 times higher for nurses who smoke than for those who don't smoke.

The rates and kinds of illnesses and disabilities that prevail in a community offer a more refined measure of the health of a population than do birth and death rates. Patterns of morbidity are determined and anticipated not only from incidence rates of reportable infectious diseases but also from prevalence rates of chronic diseases and disability; maternal-child health indices, such as percentages of pregnant women receiving adequate prenatal care; and rates of mental-health and behavioral problems, such as depression, substance abuse, and tobacco use. In the best of all possible worlds, these data would all be readily available and recorded in a format that would encourage comparability over time, between sub-population groups, and at state, national, and international levels. But this is not always the case, making it very important to know where and how to access data for a comprehensive community health assessment.

ACCESSING PUBLIC HEALTH DATA

Although information about the culture and health of a community is not always formatted in a way that will immediately answer the public health questions we may have, all levels of government are charged with collecting data about various aspects of community life, ranging from education to economic status to health. With the advances of electronic communication, we have access to more data than at any other point in history.

THE U.S. CENSUS

Mandated by the U.S. Constitution as written in 1787, the census is conducted every 10 years. Socio-demographic information, including various aspects of health and social life, is collected, analyzed, and reported for the entire United States and subdivided by states, counties, cities, towns, and census tracts.

Conducting the national census is an enormous undertaking. Although it is true that the data are less current by the time they are analyzed and reported, the census report is nevertheless very useful for showing trends over time and establishing a national database for benchmarking progress. The census data are extrapolated from a weighted representative sample. Some of the census statistics must be defined before interpretation. The unemployment rate, for example, can be subject to a wide range of definitions. The census also makes an important distinction between families and households, which is highly useful for community health purposes. Most of the census data is available on the Internet and in libraries. In addition, most states have a databank center that produces a condensed summary of each geo-political unit (that is, town, city, and county).

THE CENTERS FOR DISEASE CONTROL AND PREVENTION (CDC)

Located in Atlanta, Georgia, the mission of the CDC, an agency of the U.S. Department of Health and Human Services, is to promote health and quality of life by preventing and controlling disease, injury, and disability. The CDC is responsible for gathering information on all reportable diseases, collecting data from state health departments, and conducting and sponsoring research on various health problems in the United States. The *Morbidity and Mortality Weekly Report* (MMWR) published by the CDC summarizes information on common infectious diseases on a national level and contains news on specific outbreaks of diseases in various areas of the country (http://www.cdc.gov/mmwr/index.html). A most recent example is the CDC publication of the "Sexually Transmitted Diseases Treatment Guideline, 2015." Similar data are available on the international level from the World Health Organization (WHO).

The National Health Survey, first conducted in 1956, contains synthesized information about the state of health and health services in the United States. Using probability-sampling techniques, ongoing surveys of households permit estimates of the prevalence of specific health problems, including minor illnesses and disability. Since then, many surveys have been developed that constitute ongoing national data sets—for example, the National Health and Nutrition Examination Survey (NHANES), which measures the general health status of the total U.S. population, and the Hispanic Health and Nutrition Examination Survey (HHANES), which measures the health status of Hispanic Americans.

STATE HEALTH DEPARTMENTS

State health departments usually are a good source of relevant health data and reveal county-by-county differences in health status. They vary, however, in their requirements for reporting disease and the extent to which residents are surveyed for specific health problems. These data are particularly useful if health services are organized on a county basis. For example, in some states, records are kept on all firearms-related injuries treated in all emergency rooms. Other states may have the capacity to provide health-status indicators to local communities. Although most libraries have a government-documents department to facilitate access to these statistics, increasingly these data are available through the Internet or through computer programs developed specifically for these purposes.

LOCAL SOURCES

Birth and death registries (which also are organized by the federal government) and state, municipal, and county records on mortality and morbidity statistics are sources of current data. Schools and industries ordinarily keep records on group absenteeism, accidents, injuries, and other health problems. Many record group results of personality inventories, intelligence tests, and various screening programs as well as utilization data, such as immunization programs, counseling and education centers, and visits to the school nurse.

Records from hospitals, clinics, and other health agencies, including professional associations and healthcare voluntary associations, are yet another source of local information on population health. Unlike school and industry records, they reflect only utilization data rather than health-status data. They do not take into account all those who have a health problem (incidence and prevalence data)—only those who are receiving care. Because many people who are in need of healthcare do not access it for various reasons, utilization statistics fall short in accurately describing the level of morbidity and predicting the need for health services. Information derived from all health-provider agencies, therefore, must be supplemented with data from other sources to acquire the most comprehensive picture of the health status of a community. Local health departments may have data based on a recent assessment of health needs as a basis for local planning efforts and thus are the repository of much useful information about the health problems of a community and resources available to deal with them. The county coroner's office can be helpful in gathering data on deaths by accident, suicide, and homicide.

HEALTH SURVEYS AND EPIDEMIOLOGICAL STUDIES

National, state, and local health surveys provide even more detailed and equally important sources of data about the occurrence, distribution, and causes of current health problems. These surveys are undertaken routinely by the government; schools; hospitals; voluntary associations, such as the American Cancer Society and the American Heart Association; and universities engaged in epidemiological or health-policy research. Together, these surveys provide longitudinal and cross-sectional data on the population's health.

Although sources vary in the degree to which their information is accurate and reliable, dated or less-comprehensive information should not be dismissed, for it may be the only information available. Using imperfect information simply requires that it be identified as such and interpreted with caution. Because assessments of poorer or better community health status rely on comparisons with other communities; with state, national, and international statistics and indicators; and with other time periods, a wide range of sources must be accessed. Federal agencies that are sources of national health data sets list Internet links to state departments of health. The following section lists credible Internet sites that provide not only comprehensive data but also quick snapshots of health statistics at the international, national, and state levels. Many of these sites compile their information from the WHO and the CDC, which house global and U.S. health statistics, respectively.

INTERNET SOURCES FOR HEALTH STATISTICS

Listed in the next sections are credible and helpful resources for public health work. This is a mere sampling of the resources available.

Suggested Activity

Using Web-search tactics, identify additional information on the area in which you are working or researching.

International Health Resources

- International Agency for Research on Cancer (http://www.iarc.fr)

- International Association of Gerontology and Geriatrics (http://www.iagg.info)

- International Council of Nurses (http://www.icn.ch)

- UNAIDS (http://www.unaids.org)

- World Health Organization (http://www.who.int/en)

- World Health Organization, Ageing Topics (http://www.who.int/topics/ageing/en)

U.S. National and Governmental Health Resources

- AIDS.gov (https://www.aids.gov)

- Agency for Healthcare Research and Quality, U.S. Department of Health and Human Services (http://www.ahrq.gov)

- American Nurses Association, Policy and Advocacy (http://nursingworld.org/MainMenuCategories/ANAPoliticalPower.aspx)

- American Public Health Association (http://www.apha.org)

- Centers for Disease Control and Prevention, U.S. Department of Health and Human Services (http://www.cdc.gov)

- Centers for Disease Control and Prevention, U.S. Department of Health and Human Services, Diseases and Conditions (http://www.cdc.gov/DiseasesConditions/index.html)

- Centers for Disease Control and Prevention, U.S. Department of Health and Human Services, *Morbidity and Mortality Weekly Report* (http://www.cdc.gov/mmwr/index.html)

- Centers for Disease Control and Prevention, U.S. Department of Health and Human Services, National Center for Health Statistics (http://www.cdc.gov/nchs)

- Centers for Medicare and Medicaid Services, U.S. Department of Health and Human Services (https://www.cms.gov)

- ChildStats (http://www.childstats.gov)

- Federal Emergency Management Agency, U.S. Department of Homeland Security (http://www.fema.gov)

- HealthFinder, Office of Disease Prevention and Health Promotion, U.S. Department of Health and Human Services (http://healthfinder.gov)

- *Healthy People 2020*, Office of Disease Prevention and Health Promotion, U.S. Department of Health and Human Services (http://www.healthypeople.gov)

- Medicare (https://www.medicare.gov)

- National Cancer Institute, National Institutes of Health, U.S. Department of Health and Human Services (http://www.cancer.gov)

- National Consumer Protection Week (http://www.ncpw.gov)

- National Institutes of Health, U.S. Department of Health and Human Services (http://www.nih.gov)

- Office of Minority Health, U.S. Department of Health and Human Services (http://www.minorityhealth.hhs.gov)

- Public Health Foundation (http://www.phf.org/Pages/default.aspx)

- U.S. National Library of Medicine, National Institutes of Health, U.S. Department of Health and Human Services (https://www.nlm.nih.gov)

- Congressional Institute (http://conginst.org)

- Trust for America's Health (http://healthyamericans.org)

- U.S. Census Bureau (http://www.census.gov)

- U.S. Census Bureau, American FactFinder (http://factfinder.census.gov/faces/nav/jsf/pages/index.xhtml)

- U.S. Department of Health and Human Services (http://www.hhs.gov)

- U.S. Food and Drug Administration (http://www.fda.gov)

- Center for Food Safety and Applied Nutrition, U.S. Food and Drug Administration (http://www.fda.gov/Food/default.htm)

- U.S. White House (https://www.whitehouse.gov)

Sample U.S. State-Based Resources

- Commonwealth of Massachusetts Executive Office of Health and Human Services (http://www.mass.gov/eohhs/gov/departments/dph/)

- Illinois Health Resources (www.illinoishealthresources.org/)

- Iowa Department of Public Health (http://www.idph.iowa.gov)

- New England Alliance for Public Health Workforce Development, Health Resources and Services Administration, U.S. Department of Health and Human Services (http://bhpr.hrsa.gov/grants/publichealth/trainingcenters/about/newenglandphwd.html)

Environmental Resources

- Environmental Law Net: Laws and Regulations (www.environmentallawnet.com/lawsregs.html)

- Scorecard: The Pollution Information Site (http://scorecard.goodguide.com)

- United Nations Environment Programme (http://www.unep.org)

- U.S. Environmental Protection Agency (http://www3.epa.gov)

- Envirofacts Data Warehouse, U.S. Environmental Protection Agency (http://catalog.data.gov/dataset/envirofacts-data-warehouse)

- Superfund Program, U.S. Environmental Protection Agency (http://www2.epa.gov/superfund)

- Learn About Water, U.S. Environmental Protection Agency (http://water.epa.gov)

- World Resources Institute (http://www.wri.org)

- World Wildlife Fund—Conservation (http://www.panda.org)

Population Resources
- Population Institute (https://www.populationinstitute.org)

- Population Reference Bureau (http://www.prb.org)

- United Nations Population Fund (http://www.unfpa.org)

Topic-Specific Resources
- Administration on Aging, U.S. Department of Health and Human Services (http://www.aoa.gov)

- American Cancer Society (http://www.cancer.org)

- The John A. Hartford Foundation (http://www.jhartfound.org)

- Medscape (http://www.medscape.com)

- National Breast Cancer Foundation, Inc. (http://www.nationalbreastcancer.org)

- OncoLink (http://www.oncolink.org/index.cfm?)

- ABCD: After Breast Cancer Diagnosis (http://www.y-me.org)

CULTURALLY INFORMED COMMUNITY HEALTH ANALYSIS

In community/public health practice, cultural information and health information cannot be considered separately. The ethnographic cultural inquiry of the community provides the context in which community strengths (cultural capital) are better understood, and the health risks and problems, identified through epidemiological research, are interpreted, prioritized, addressed, and ameliorated through using and building cultural capital.

Illnesses, injuries, safety problems, and unhealthy behaviors are better understood by examining them in the sociocultural milieu where they occur and interact. High rates of cancer, for example, could be related to the presence of a nuclear energy plant and faulty methods of waste disposal in one community, while in another it could be linked to the age distribution of the population. Both communities have a high rate of cancer, but plans for effective prevention, advocacy, and system-level intervention must vary according to local conditions and cultural capital.

In community/public health practice, four basic questions need to be asked of all information acquired in our community culture inquiry and health assessment:

- **How does the community information vary with time? For example:**

  a. In the culture inquiry: How does the number and quality of housing units compare with the previous 5 or 10 years?

  b. In the health assessment: How does the current incidence of elder abuse and neglect compare with the previous 5 and 10 years?

- **How does the community information compare with similar communities and with local, state, national, and international findings? For example:**

  a. In the culture inquiry: How does the proportion of residents over 65 compare with the proportion of those individuals at the state, national, and international levels?

  b. In the health assessment: How does the community's rate of Alzheimer's disease and other types of dementia compare at the county, state, national, and international levels?

- **How does the information in the various categories of the culturally informed community assessment relate to information in other categories? For example:**

  a. In the culture inquiry: How are community programs serving older adults related to politics or economic factors?

b. In the health assessment: How are disparities in elder services linked to time, place, population characteristics, and social organization?

■ **What are the implications of the community information for health and health-care?** For example:

a. In the culture inquiry: What are the implications of a tourist-based economy for the health of elder community residents?

b. In the health assessment: What are the implications of air pollution on the health of elder community residents?

THE PRACTICE PROJECT

By now, you have learned that being responsible for the health of a whole community is an awesome undertaking and differs greatly from caring for an individual in clinical practice. It requires a different kind of knowledge and skill set to help communities build capacity for health. Chapters 1–3 explored the unique history, assumptions, ethics, values, and strategies that are central to community/public health nursing. Equipped with this arsenal of concepts and knowledge, you are ready to begin the exciting work of leading change in healthcare—not just treating disease, patient by patient, but creating health and ensuring social justice and equity. This chapter is about your role in the community. It is about building relationships with community residents and institutions.

It is about collecting, organizing, and managing relevant information about your community so that you will make culturally informed decisions and work with community partners to create an achievable and sustainable healthy community agenda.

CHAPTER 4 OBJECTIVES

- Know the significance of your demeanor and behavior in building a strong relationship with your community, and apply it accordingly.

- Organize and manage the information you acquire about your community.

- Understand and apply the culturally informed community nursing practice process.

■ Develop analytical skills through comparisons within your community, with other communities, and within the context in which your community sits (e.g., county, state, and national levels).

ENTERING AND ENGAGING: NEW ROLES, NEW RELATIONSHIPS

It is liberating to think critically and yet be open, flexible, and nonjudgmental. This enables you to see the community not just through your own lens but also through the eyes of community members. For example, when first entering a small Caribbean village, students did not know where to purchase food or water. There were no identifiable grocery stores or supermarkets. After living in the village a short time, however, they found there was an abundance of food. Growing and selling food was a major cottage industry for villagers, occurring on every street and byway and from villagers' homes to large roadside markets on specific days of the week.

Working with a community can be challenging, even frustrating, especially if you have been accustomed to being organized in your classes and "in control" of hospital patient encounters in clinical practice. Acute care settings are the "turf" of healthcare providers who "own" and control that setting. Conversely, patients lying in bed in an acute care hospital have no control over who walks in the room and no choice regarding the nurse caring for them. Now you are in an unfamiliar community, "owned" by residents and businesspeople who may or may not agree to follow your advice or even to meet with you. This is why relationship building is so important in community health practice: The rapport you establish in the community will yield unlimited opportunities to build community partnerships, think creatively, and capture the vision of community health.

The realization that community/public health work cannot be done alone, nor can it be accomplished solely by healthcare professionals, is the starting point for public health practice. Community/public health nursing work is not limited to caring for community-based patients in specific nursing services or public health agencies. Creating a healthy public requires good communication and solid connections throughout the entire community, including legislators, educators, faith leaders, media personnel, and other high-profile community actors. Organizational partners representing various sectors of the community—civic societies, local businesses, faith-based institutions, schools and universities—and grassroots groups, such as "Citizens for Social Action," are essential to getting the job done. Local healthcare education programs are important collaborators, bringing faculty and students to practice and learn, while at the same time doing something really important for the communities that you study.

This relationship-building work is not "in addition to" your public health work—it *is* public health work and is the foundation of your success in building healthy communities. Therefore, as you are doing your assessment, it is important to keep a running list of all community members with whom you and your team have spoken about the project, their contact information, and their interest and/or possible involvement in the community health project.

Suggested Activity

Construct a community partnership log:

Name	Contact Information	Interest	Notes

CONSIDERING DEMEANOR AND DEPORTMENT

Attire, grooming, and manners all form a presentation of yourself that leaves a lasting first impression. Because uniforms and scrubs generally are not appropriate or required in community health practice, dressing professionally and appropriately requires attention. Appropriateness is determined by the purpose and context in which you are participating. If, for example, you are invited to an executive or community board meeting, it is appropriate to wear dignified and modest clothing—no shorts, T-shirts, denim, sneakers, or dangly jewelry. Instead, choose trousers, skirts, sweaters, jackets, and suits. If, however, you are working with children at the local neighborhood playground, just the opposite is true. Dressing for the occasion is just another form of communication that will go a long way in establishing your credibility with all sectors of the community.

Prior to meeting with community members and partners, it is important to pre-

Suggested Activity

With your team members, do the following:

- Draft a message to the manager of the local recreation center, requesting a meeting to tour the facility and to learn about community programs. Ask others to read and critique your email regarding its ability to effectively and clearly communicate your intended purpose and needs.

- Explore and discuss professional strategies for following up with additional communication if you do not receive a response in what you consider to be a timely manner. How do you determine a "timely manner"?

- Draft another message to the recreation center manager to thank him or her for the tour of the facility, the overview of the community programs the center offers, and the center manager's interest in working with you.

- Discuss ways to maintain effective communication with community members/partners, such as, "How would you prefer to communicate (phone, email, contacting secretary, etc.)?"

- Discuss events or issues that can cause problems with communication in the example above and strategies to address these problems to maintain positive communications. For example, it may be difficult to have uninterrupted meeting time with the manager of a busy recreation center with many employees. Suggest that the meeting occur toward the end of the day or outside work hours to avoid interruption.

pare for the meeting. Do a little research in advance you so that you know something about the community members/partners (e.g., look up their names and professional positions online) and have a clear and succinct purpose for the meeting prior to making the appointment. Introduce yourself and team members by first and last name, including your university/college affiliation, program, and professor. Professional dress will depend on the purpose and context of the meeting. Use professional etiquette, including acknowledging the receptionist, offering the appropriate greeting (e.g., handshake, head nod, etc.), waiting to be invited to sit, and requesting to take notes during the meeting. At the conclusion, briefly synthesize the key points of the meeting, thank them for visiting with you, and let them know when you will be following up with them (as appropriate).

After visits with community members, it is important to follow up and thank them for their interest and/or support. Whether you send a note, phone call, or email, appropriate etiquette regarding the use of titles and salutations is critical. If you are in doubt, consult online resources that offer guidelines for professional formal communication.

ENGAGING IN EFFECTIVE TEAM MEMBER RELATIONSHIPS

As you enter the community, you represent not only yourself but also your school, faculty members, preceptors, the nursing profession, and others who are engaged in this line of work. As an exemplary ambassador for health and nursing, you will continue to strengthen the reputation of your team, increasing its effectiveness. Your team works *interdependently* as a small health coalition, as members cooperate with (not compete against) each other to accomplish a common goal. It is to each student's benefit to help one another and to engage in positive group process skills. As you continue to work in your community health team, it is important to discuss, reaffirm, and, if necessary, renegotiate for consensus on your group norms. Determine each of your team member's strengths and how he or she can be best used to accomplish goals. Identify expectations, such as meeting attendance, communications, timeliness of the work, format of the work, and formative group feedback, so that all members are clear as to expectations and outcomes.

For example, a student who enjoys writing may take the lead on organizing the different documents, whereas another student who enjoys working with cloud-based technology may commit to organizing the community assessment and taking the lead on putting a shared worksite together. Other students may feel better suited to taking the lead on the literature searches, contacting and following up with key informants, or being responsible for organizing the group meeting agendas and keeping meeting minutes.

Suggested Activity

As a team with a common goal, meet with one another to:

- Discuss parameters of when, how often, and where you will meet.
- Set standards and expectations for the group process that all agree to.
- Do an Internet search and identify the format the team will use for team meeting agendas and minutes.
- Discuss how you will communicate with a team member who is not abiding by the team agreement.
- Construct a written agreement, with all members signing the document, to ensure mutual understanding of what is expected.

ORGANIZING AND MANAGING THE COMMUNITY INFORMATION

Assessing the whole community as a unit for nursing care may seem daunting at first, especially for nursing students or new nurses who are entering an area as a community/public health nurse for the first time. You are meeting new people, collecting much information from various sources, reading local newspapers, following community blogs, discovering a variety of social organizations that serve all or a select group of members of the community, learning about community events, and beginning to better understand the strengths and issues prevalent in the community. It is common to feel overwhelmed and sometimes frustrated with managing all the information. Sometimes assessment data are simply not available, and other times communication barriers with community partners cause efforts to flounder. You may feel you are "swimming" in information and do not understand where your efforts will lead, fearing you are not on the right track or that you do not know what you are doing. (These feelings are common and *likely mean that you are doing the culturally informed assessment correctly*, because you are remaining open to learning about and from the community.) Training to move beyond prejudgments (often unconscious beliefs) is important and may require continuous reminders between team members. A personal Community Practice Notebook facilitates development of openness to cultural information and an awareness of your own biases. These data will then better inform the community health field notes that you share with your team members.

Communities may seem big and diverse and outside your control to capture and use information that will give you a clear understanding of their cultures. But getting to know the culture and health of your community is not only possible but also enjoyable when you systematically organize your observations, experiences, and interviews. This process is similar to how you learned to conduct a history and physical on an individual patient, only now your client is the community. By following this method, you will be able to speak to what you have discovered in your community assessment so that the relationships you form and the information you collect are useful for developing community health programming.

Suggested Activity

With a personal and confidential Community Practice Notebook, track community observations and interactions. Examples of things to include in a personal Community Practice Notebook include newspaper clippings, flyers, articles, and other documents collected in the process of entering and learning about your community. These data then will be organized according to the culturally informed community health assessment described in Chapters 5 and 6.

Personal Community Practice Notebook

Date _____ Time _____ Event _____

Goals for this culturally informed community assessment activity:

Description of the activity:

Write about and draw diagrams to describe the experience you had in the community. Include the place, people, and activities that you observed and/or participated in. Do not judge the experience or evaluate it. Describe it so that when you read through this description at a later time, you will have a clear picture and understanding of the experience. If you are doing this correctly, it will take time and thought to complete the entry. Details are important in this step, because you will use some of this description to complete your culturally informed community health assessment. After your description, include the following:

- **Professional interpretation:** As you record information about the community, also note your initial interpretation based on the literature that you have read, course work, class discussion, research, practice models, and your thinking about the experience.

- **Personal reactions:** Describe your response to the community and the people you have met. From your perspective, what went well, what did not go well, and how do you "feel" about the experience? This information will not be included in the community assessment but rather serve as a way of helping you check your own biases.

Plans for next community practice activity:

Include the following:

- **Professional:** Describe areas that you want to assess further, resources or collaborative relationships you will explore, community models, programs and interventions, objectives and goals, and the effectiveness of and/or necessary modifications to the strategic plan.

- **Personal:** What went well, what did not go so well, or what did you feel uncomfortable with? Describe how you might handle the situation in the future and resources you will explore for your own growth and understanding. This information will not be included in the community assessment but rather serve as a way of helping you cope with challenges.

This is a personal and confidential notebook. Your identify and identities of community members in the notebook should be protected in case of loss or theft.

Discuss with your team members how each of you will use your personal Community Practice Notebook to then organize the *team's* community health field notes (e.g., identifying a place where all the team members' field notes are kept, synthesizing the weekly activities into one set of field notes, etc.).

Community Health Field Notes

Time	Date and Event	Index	Personal Comments	Follow Up

As you collect this extensive community information, it is helpful to take a larger view of the culturally informed community health assessment. This assessment is organized as a 2 X 3 framework that helps organize your thinking, writing, and analysis. *Community Culture Inquiry* and *Community Health Assessment* are the two larger categories that are then systematically assessed in the three areas of *Environment*, *Population*, and *Social Organization*.

	Environment	Population	Social Organization
Culture Inquiry			
Health Assessment			

In Chapters 5 and 6, the content and structure of the community culture inquiry and community health assessments, respectively, are explained and clarified for you. As with the health assessments of individuals you perform in clinical practice, not all components of the assessment tool will be relevant to all communities, so do not worry about filling in every category of information. Furthermore, as you learned in Chapter 3, communities are long-term "clients" with histories that may span decades and even centuries. In the limited time you will have to learn about your community client (e.g., one semester), it is not possible to collect information about every aspect of culture and health. Collecting information about a "living" community is a continuous and an unpredictable component of public health practice. In the event of a hurricane, for example, the community could change significantly in a single day. Conversely, it may take decades for a community to transform from an agricultural to a tourist economy. The assessment tool is simply a useful and tested way to outline and categorize data about the community to easily access information for planning and intervention.

Culturally Informed Community Health Assessment Tool
Community Culture Inquiry

I. Physical Environment of a Community
   A. Spatial dimensions
      1. Boundaries, size, and distribution
      2. Regional position
      3. Geophysical and climate factors
      4. Land use
      5. Housing
      6. Transportation
      7. Communication
      8. Mental maps
   B. Temporal (yearly, monthly, weekly, daily working calendars and schedules)
      1. Community history
      2. Cyclical population movement
      3. Economic cycles
      4. Psychological cycles
      5. Cyclical crises

II. Population of a Community
   A. Total population (size, density, distribution)
   B. Temporary subpopulations
   C. Biological composition (age and sex)
   D. Ethnic and racial groups
   E. Occupation, income, and education level
   F. Residential and household characteristics

III. Social Organization of a Community
   A. Community institutions
      1. Economic
      2. Government, politics, and law enforcement
      3. Domestic
      4. Religion
      5. Education
      6. Recreation
      7. Voluntary
   B. Horizontal stratification
   C. Vertical segmentation

Community Health Assessment

I. Environmental Health
   A. Outdoor air quality
   B. Surface- and ground-water quality
   C. Food contamination
   D. Toxic substances and hazardous-waste management
      1. Solid waste
      2. Sewage
      3. Radioactive waste
      4. Chemicals and pesticides
   E. Noise pollution
   F. Disease vectors
   G. Preparedness
   H. Crime
   I. Accidents
   J. Homes and communities

K. Community buildings

L. Energy management

M. Global health

II. Population Health

    A. Infectious diseases

    B. Chronic diseases

    C. Chronic disability

    D. Behavioral and mental health

    E. Maternal, infant, and child health

    F. Early and middle childhood health

    G. Adolescent health

    H. Older adult health

    I. Lesbian, gay, bisexual, and transgender health

    J. Occupational safety and health

    K. Population health behaviors

III. Health Care Organization: Institutional and Ideological Dimensions

    A. Health workforce such as:

        1. Nursing

        2. Medical

        3. Dental

        4. Social work

        5. Mental health

        6. Nutrition

        7. Optical/audiology

        8. Therapies, such as physical, occupational, speech

    B. Public health agencies

        1. Health departments

        2. Personal healthcare agencies such as:

            a. Hospitals ("health centers")

   b. Nursing homes, extended care facilities, assisted living

   c. Home health agencies

   d. Freestanding ambulatory facilities

  3. Health planning agencies

C. Public health financing

  1. Third-party payers

   a. Commercial

   b. Government

  2. Self-pay

  3. Charity

  4. Public assistance

D. Health values and beliefs

  1. Customs

  2. Traditions

  3. Values

E. Indigenous and alternative health systems

As you continue to collect information, organize it into each of the categories in this culturally informed community health assessment. Initially, you may find it most helpful to include bulleted information (e.g., words, maps, photos, and statistics) with the associated citations and/or links to the information. Because a community is ever-changing, you will discover that community assessment is a dynamic and ongoing process. As you have sufficient information for each category, review and analyze the bulleted information and write a description of each category. Carefully note your valid and reliable Internet links so that you have access to information online that will be regularly updated; this will help you create a "living document" from which to pull your information.

As you perform the assessment, foster a spirit of flexibility and use critical thinking when gathering information. Each of your communities and target communities is different. As such, it may not be possible to identify or locate all the information included in the outline, or you may believe the information requested does not relate to your community. It is also possible that you may identify information that you think is important to include but is not listed as an assessment parameter. The outline provided is a framework, so feel free to modify it according to the needs of your community. It just needs to make sense.

Suggested Activity

Do the following:

- Use the culturally informed community health assessment tool as an outline to create or refine your own document for the Community Culture Inquiry with the identified "Physical Environment," "Population," and "Social Organization" headings and appropriate subheadings under each of these categories (Chapter 5).

- Create the second section of the document to include the Community Health Assessment "Environmental Health," "Population Health," and "Healthcare Organization" headings with the appropriate subheadings (Chapter 6).

- Create a third section of the document to include "Planning" and the implications for community healthcare: the list of community health issues evident in the culturally informed community assessment (Chapter 7).

- Create a fourth section of the document to include "Programming/Interventions," "Programming Outcomes," and "Planning Updates or Next Steps" (Chapter 8).

UNDERSTANDING THE COMMUNITY INFORMATION

After you have the appropriate categories for your community assessment described, you are ready to analyze and synthesize the community information. Look at your community information again and ask questions about:

- How the information about this community varies by time

- How the information varies with other similar communities

- How the information varies within the different categories of the assessment

It is often helpful to create a matrix or table or to draw a diagram to help you analyze the information. Feel free to be creative as you consider what the information is telling you about the culture and health of the community. This analysis will then provide the evidence for you to begin to identify implications for health and healthcare.

Seasonal Crime Incidence in Different Regions of the Community

	North Side	South Side	West Side	East Side
Winter				
Spring				
Summer				
Autumn				

A useful strategy to organize the implications for health and healthcare is to use a community nursing diagnosis framework. You can use the NANDA Nursing Diagnosis format or the Omaha System and/or modify an *individual* focused nursing diagnosis so that it accurately represents a *community or population* focus. Based on the evidence from your community culture inquiry and health assessments, formulate possible community health diagnoses using the following process:

■ Identify risks to the health of this community.

■ Identify the segments of the community affected by these risks.

■ Identify potential short- and long-term culture-based responses to the risk.

These diagnoses or descriptive statements are essential to communicating with your key constituents and focusing on culturally informed (evidence-based) issues and solutions. This strategy also helps distinguish the *community's* problems from the *agency's* problems.

FRAMING THE CULTURALLY INFORMED NURSING PRACTICE PROJECT PROCESS

The community assessment is foundational to creating a healthy community agenda and engaging in culturally informed community action. Before beginning the assessment, let's take a few minutes to review the whole process and demonstrate how you will write up a synthesis of your community (see Figure 4.1).

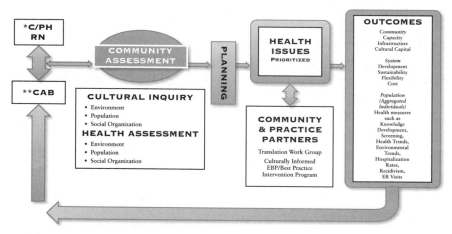

* **C/PH RN:** Community/Public Health Registered Nurse
* **CAB:** Community Advisory Board

Figure 4.1   The culturally informed community nursing practice process.
Copyright © Skemp, L., & Peacock, M., 2015. Used with permission.

In Figure 4.1, the community/public health nursing student (or C/PH RN) and the team of other nursing students identify a community with the assistance of the community/public health nursing instructor. The instructor helps the nurses make contact with key members of the community, who will introduce them to other key community members and the educational purpose of the community/public health nursing experience. Some of these persons may already be on a community advisory board (CAB), although membership will likely be formed and modified over the course of doing the assessment and working with community members.

The *community assessment* process is organized to provide a straightforward 2 X 3 framework in which to collect and organize the information about the community. This framework includes working with community partners (the developing community advisory board) as you conduct the cultural inquiry of the community (the environment, people, and how they organize themselves) and the health assessment of the community (the health of the environment, the health of the people, and healthcare organizations). Many communities may have an *overarching healthy community agenda* in place; some may not. In either case, this is a critical piece of information to integrate into the community assessment. The cultural inquiry helps you better *identify and understand* the health issues and the *cultural capital* (people, institutions, and resources) to address the issue.

With your community partners (e.g., the CAB), you then begin planning to (a) identify and prioritize the key health issues and (b) determine the community and interdisciplinary practice partners best able to help translate the evidence-based and/or best practices into culturally informed programming to improve the outcomes.

Here is an example of a culturally informed description of the community of Bonterre:

> Bonterre is a rural community located in the farm belt of the Midwest. The population of 2,500 people is mostly engaged in grain agriculture production and a small meatpacking industry. These industries have been the lifeblood of the community since before it was officially founded in 1892 by a small group of German settlers seeking political freedom. Bonterre's population grew rapidly

in the first 100 years due to the railroads, stabilized, and recently decreased as young people migrated to Minneapolis and Chicago. The population has again increased with the recruitment of immigrants to work in the local meatpacking industry. There is a small K–8 school, a library, three churches, and a nurse-run clinic—high school, acute care, public health department, etc., are regionalized in larger towns and cities. With the continued outmigration of young people, many of the farms are now worked by migrants during the farming season. There is a high population of elders (18%), and many middle-age persons commute to nearby cities for work.

Because of the population skew toward older adults, chronic diseases, such as diabetes, have become an increasing problem. Furthermore, because people of Latino heritage carry a higher risk for and incidence of diabetes, the migrant population is also in need of health promotion and disease prevention. The increasing incidence of diabetes in the older population and more recently in the new immigrant population has increased rates of worker absenteeism, clinic visits, and hospitalizations. The regional health department does not provide elder or diabetes services. The nurse has identified a 20% rise in clinic visits associated with diabetes and diabetes-related foot problems, but no programs for foot care or diabetes-related foot problems are available. This lack has resulted in an increase in the rate of lower-extremity amputations over the last 5 years, disability rates, clinic visits and costs, and loss of work time. The problem is particularly relevant in the immigrant Latino community. There are significant cultural differences between the historically European population and the immigrant Latino population, including language, religious beliefs and practices, customs, and values.

Thus, two community and practice partner translation workgroups were formed. A best practice program to provide foot care was agreed upon within each of the workgroups and then translated into appropriate programming in each of the communities. For example, the programming for the Latino group occurred at the local Catholic church, and a female community member was trained to provide the programming. Programming for the community of European heritage took place at the local senior center, and training included several volunteers from the health department.

Outcomes included increased community capacity (e.g., increased cultural capital by training members of the Latino community to run the program and developed programming at a senior center), system outcomes (e.g., decreased costs of lost work and worker turnover and decreased hospitalizations far from home), and population outcomes (e.g., increased screening of persons with diabetes-related foot problems).

Ongoing strategic planning then included development of policies for nurse-led primary care reimbursement to serve these (essentially invisible) communities and a proposal writing team to seek out funding to continue the programs. These outcomes then influenced how the community/public health nurse and the CAB continued to assess and manage the issues within the larger healthy community agenda to promote equity and social justice. The success of the foot care programs led the community/public health nurse to visit with the director of the regional public health department to discuss the development of a community action plan to specifically address the needs of the older population and the new immigrants. Recognizing the diverse cultural differences in the communities served, the coalition members included elder and middle-age Latino and Caucasian community members who were served at the foot-clinic programs, church leaders, and the nurse at the nurse-run clinic. They took the lead in planning to incorporate these issues into the larger regional healthy community agenda.

SITUATIONS TO HELP ASSESS A COMMUNITY

Reflecting on other examples of community health situations can help you as you begin to perform a community assessment. As you read through the following vignettes, identify the issues and reflect on what was done well and what could be done differently. Which components of a culturally informed assessment are present and which components are needed to better understand the community? How would you write up the description of the different scenarios to follow a systematic, culturally informed approach? These situations help you see your own community in ways that may not be readily apparent and remain open to what your community has to tell you.

TEENVILLE AND OBEVILLE: OBESITY AND TEEN PREGNANCY

In a rural U.S. county of approximately 34,000 persons, statistics revealed that rates of teen pregnancy, sexually transmitted diseases (STDs), and obesity exceeded rates across the region and the state. In one community of approximately 1,500 persons, which we will call "Teenville," the community/public health nurse was new to the community. To begin to address this identified "problem," he invited members of the community to come together to discuss the community health concern, recommending that the school nurse provide birth-control information and condoms in her office. He believed the meeting went well. Community members attended and listened to his plan. Assuming that the community members who met together wanted to keep up the community health improvement momentum and be part of his community action plan, he gathered names and contact information so that he could follow up with them after the meeting.

When no one responded to his follow-up communications, he reached out to a nearby college of nursing for assistance with brainstorming new strategies on ways to reduce the teen-pregnancy rate. Working in partnership, a team of nursing students conducted a culturally informed community assessment that included attitudes about health education and teen pregnancy and explored the resources available to the community. Visiting with members of the community (many of whom had attended the earlier meeting), they were able to learn that the community values were largely conservative and that the community's members "did not agree that teen pregnancy" was an issue, despite the statistics. They were offended at the idea of condoms and in particular at providing them to their children in the school nurse's office. They wanted the school to present an "abstinence-only" health program. However, members of the community advisory board did have concerns about the older citizens in their community and explained that a better use of the community/public health nurse's time and effort was to go to the senior citizen lunch site, take blood pressures, and educate people on ways to age more safely in their own homes.

In another small community of 1,000 persons in the same county, "Obeville," the community/public health nurse was working with university nursing students on conducting a culturally informed community assessment. Like the community of "Teenville," the community advisory board did not believe teen pregnancy or STDs were a problem. Rather, they decided to focus on a community exercise program because of the high obesity rate and a concern about the recent fatal heart attack of a very respected middle-age member of the community. A community exercise program was developed in the community during the first year. Community members then took over management of the exercise program, and the local school requested that the nursing students help them create a similar program for grades K–12. Over the next three semesters, this developed into four programs: (a) community wide, (b) grades K–3, (c) grades 4–8, and (d) grades 9–12. The following semester, the advisory board requested that the community/ public health nurse and the next group of students evaluate the high teen-pregnancy and STD rates and recommend programs to address them.

These community/public health nurses and students discovered through the Community Culture Inquiry and Health Assessment that, although teen pregnancy, STDs, and obesity were statistically significant health problems, the primary concerns of community members must be considered: in Teenville, the needs of the large elder community, and in Obeville, the obesity rate and cardiac health concerns. This consideration was essential to establishing trust and credibility with local community members. As trust and credibility were established, the community members became more open to addressing more sensitive community issues.

Suggested Activity

Answer the following:

- What are the key issues in this vignette?
- What was done well in this situation?
- Considering a culturally informed approach:
    a. What additional information do you need?
    b. What could be done differently in this situation?

URBANVILLE: HOMELESSNESS IN OUR COMMUNITIES

In Urbanville, a community of 120,000 located near the crossroads of several large interstate highways, the problem of homelessness had been growing each year. The community, known for its relative prosperity and job growth, magnetically attracted individuals fleeing generational poverty and urban violence as well as people from other communities with few jobs and limited low-income housing. The number of people who came to Urbanville began as a slow trickle, but as the generosity and liberal-minded spirit of the community became more widely known, the number of people who came for assistance increased each year.

Some church members banded together to provide a patchwork of supportive services for these new community members: a makeshift shelter, some food and clothing. Local agencies grew up around this shelter and its growing population: a free health clinic and free meal site. If a person had a significant health need, a local visiting nurse would visit and provide care. The shelter had dedicated volunteers and low-paid staff yet did a remarkable job of providing basic services to the people in need. Other community opinions began to emerge: Some members protested and wanted outreach efforts to stop so that the homeless population might decrease by going elsewhere, thus helping maintain the community's self-image. Nonetheless, over the course of 20 years, the number of homeless people grew, as did the resources to help them. A purpose-built homeless shelter was constructed, although not without some community dissonance. The needs of a vulnerable population were not met "perfectly," but they were addressed in a spirit of compassion. Urbanville could be considered a healthy place, and efforts to expand services and programs to have healthier people are ongoing. Sustaining these efforts requires ongoing caring, commitment, and community partnerships.

Suggested Activity

Answer the following:

- What are the key issues in this vignette?

- What was done well in this situation?

- Considering a culturally informed approach:

  a. What additional information do you need?

  b. What could be done differently in this situation?

SANIVILLE: WALKING FOR WATER, THE NEW GLOBAL GOLD

A community/public health nurse was working with a nongovernmental organization (NGO) in a developing community. She had been requested to conduct a culturally informed community assessment of the rural area village. NGO staffers were very successful in getting to know community leaders and addressing many of the community's health issues and needs, including sanitation, immunization, malaria prevention, safe childbirth, and family planning, to name a few. Addressing sanitation by providing toilet facilities was a high priority. This program required community "buy-in" in concept and practice. Community representatives were actively engaged in choosing the type of public toilets and assisted in building the facilities.

In some communities, there was good uptake and use of the new toilets; in other communities, however, the toilets were not used. In assessing the environment, population, and how community members organized themselves, much was learned about uptake by comparing different communities. For example, in one community where the toilet facilities were not being used, the community members, particularly the women, continued to use the wooded area to toilet. This made perfect sense when one better understood the culture. First, the women had to walk long distances every day to fetch water from the local well, and so they preferred to use this water for cooking and other uses rather than to flush and clean the toilet. Second, women in the village spent most of their time in and surrounding the home. Typically, the women did not walk about the village unattended by a man. Quite simply, the morning toilet in the wooded area with the other women was an opportunity to interact with one another, and the women did not want to go alone to the more isolated toilet facility, as it was not perceived to be safe for them.

Suggested Activity

Answer the following:

- What are the key issues in this vignette?
- What was done well in this situation?
- Considering a culturally informed approach:
  - a.   What additional information do you need?
  - b.   What could be done differently in this situation?

INDUSTRYVILLE: HIDDEN POPULATIONS WITHIN COMMUNITIES

An *industry* is a community with shared values, characteristics, and/or interests that unite its members. For example, nursing students worked with an occupational health nurse in an industry that was known in the region for its good salaries, positive work environment, and diverse workforce of more than 20,000 people. Job roles at this industry included professionals with desk jobs, healthcare providers, maintenance staff and groundkeepers, food servers, and other ancillary support workers. Educational preparation of the employees ranged from some employees' possessing advanced graduate education to some having less than a high school education. Although most employees spoke English as their primary language, some immigrants and refugees from diverse regions across the globe spoke minimal English. Most community assessment information could be completed using data collected by the employer, supplemented with the knowledge that employees commuted from rural and urban communities up to 1.5 hours away.

In addition to being a desirable employer that brought many jobs to the region, the industry was also unique in its commitment to the health of its employees: It offered a busy occupational health program that provided a variety of health screenings as well as assessment and treatment of work-related injuries, plus an employee wellness service and health promotion program for its workers. The most valued resource was the generous health insurance benefit, yet some pockets of employees were not accessing these resources. The nursing students engaged in a culturally informed community health assessment and discovered that two sub-groups of workers had needs that were not being sufficiently addressed:

- The maintenance and groundskeeping workers were often too busy to attend health-related events.

- A pool of part-time employees did not work at least half-time, so they did not qualify for health insurance or health-promotion services available to full-time employees.

This information was shared with an occupational health services team, and a plan for improved community action to address these health gaps was developed.

Suggested Activity

Answer the following:

- What are the key issues in this vignette?
- What was done well in this situation?
- Considering a culturally informed approach:
    - a.   What additional information do you need?
    - b.   What could be done differently in this situation?

NEIGHBORVILLE: NEIGHBORHOOD-BY-NEIGHBORHOOD

Much can be learned by looking at how communities have coped in the past. For example, after experiencing the devastation and uncertainty with the 9/11 destruction of the Twin Towers and then watching the lack of public health preparedness during the acute phase of Hurricane Katrina, community health departments were asking what they needed to do to best prepare for potential disasters. One urban community made a concerted effort to identify those homebound elders who may be at risk during a disaster. The health department conducted a public campaign to encourage elder citizens to sign up on a "disaster list" so that, in the event of a catastrophe, someone could help them evacuate. Although various forms of social media, home health, and other venues were used, the response was poor, with fewer than 50 persons agreeing to be identified. The county health department did not have the resources to go door to door and asked whether the community/public health nursing students could advance this project.

Over the next three semesters, the community/public health nursing students engaged in a culturally informed community assessment in the area of the city where many of the elders lived. Coming to understand that this area of the city was composed of well-established neighborhoods, they then developed smaller teams of students to conduct a culturally informed assessment of the neighborhood blocks, meeting key community leaders and learning about the best mechanisms to communicate with elders about the community health issue. Issues were identified, such as elder community members' fear of being forced to leave their homes and not being allowed to return, and the lack of resources for them to evacuate with their pets. Strategic plans were developed, information programs held throughout the neighborhoods, a door-to-door (neighbor to neighbor) intervention developed, the disaster policy refined, and the disaster list created. This plan was tested a few years later when a disaster occurred in the area: All homebound elders (and their pets) were successfully assisted to other areas of safe housing.

Suggested Activity

Answer the following:

- What are the key issues in this vignette?
- What was done well in this situation?
- Considering a culturally informed approach:
    a.   What additional information do you need?
    b.   What could be done differently in this situation?

STUDENTVILLE: COMMUNITY AND ISOLATION

In a large university community with a growing international student population, opportunities for international students to engage with domestic students and the larger community were limited and complicated by language and cultural barriers. Although the campus offered resources for international students, their needs were invisible. An international student who became interested in mental health concerns from her psychology classes created an outreach event for international students that focused on ways to reduce their feelings of isolation. This program led a community/public health nurse and nursing students to conduct a culturally informed community assessment that included working in partnership with the international student to survey the different groups of international students to find out what they knew about mental health, mental illness, and available mental health services on campus. A survey revealed that the international students had various understandings about the concept of mental health, stigmas associated with mental health, and no knowledge that mental health services were available to them. These somewhat hidden communities of people were identified, and interventions were developed that promoted awareness of mental health topics for the international students and the providers, thereby promoting more access to appropriate resources to help the international students deal with stress and isolation. Future plans were discussed regarding ways for international students to more intentionally engage with domestic students to further reduce their magnified feelings of social isolation.

Suggested Activity

Answer the following:

- What are the key issues in this vignette?
- What was done well in this situation?
- Considering a culturally informed approach:
  a. What additional information do you need?
  b. What could be done differently in this situation?

DATAVILLE: COMMUNITY BELIEFS, UNDERSTANDINGS, AND DATA

The community/public health nursing students and faculty had worked closely with the administrator of a local community center for a couple of years. The center was a well-established community intervention to provide Section 8 housing to those in need. A recent influx of immigrants and refugees had come to this community. Each group of community/public health nursing students updated the culturally informed community assessment with members of the advisory board. The advisory board included leaders from the immigrant and refugee community, the administrator of the center, faculty, and healthcare providers. Issues had been identified and programming begun in a variety of areas, such as "interviewing for success," "transportation," "stress management and coping," and "diabetes prevention and management." A group of community/public health nursing students and the advisory board members had identified a new area to focus on: providing access to medications. Some of the immigrant/refugee children were being diagnosed with attention deficit disorder and prescribed medications. However, their family members could not afford these medications, so the students decided to create programming to provide access to these medications.

Although observational data about the problem were provided by family members, by teachers from the schools where the children attended, and by members of the community center, the issue was not sufficiently data-driven and lacked an integration of the analysis of the history of the community and family system. Many of the immigrant and refugee families had come from war-torn areas and suffered unimaginable traumas. Additionally, the immigrants and refugees had an extended family system in which everyone in their community was responsible for the upbringing of the children, not solely their mothers or fathers. As such, data about the children being unruly on the playgrounds and in the classroom were related to parenting and schoolroom behavior expectations in the United States, not a diagnosed illness.

Rather than providing medication, programming facilitated an understanding of expectations for the children and parents in the various community settings. Teachers were also educated about the history of the community, the types of school systems the children had come from, and this group's parenting styles. The community stress and coping program was also better tailored to meet the needs of community members. Mismanagement of a community issue that could have caused harm was averted.

Suggested Activity

Do the following:

- What are the key issues in this vignette?
- What was done well in this situation?
- Considering a culturally informed approach:
    a. What additional information do you need?
    b. What could be done differently in this situation?

This chapter has discussed how information that is collected and organized using the culturally informed community health assessment process and tools will build a foundation for community partnerships and community action. You are now ready to begin your assessment, which is one of the first steps in planning for and building community capacity for health.

DISCOVERING THE CULTURE OF YOUR COMMUNITY

Culture is not just about ethnicity. Rather, it is about the way in which a community uses space and time, its lifeways, and the manners in which people are organized and interact. It also includes the ways in which health is promoted, illness is prevented, and care is provided. From a systematic examination of the community's culture, we begin to identify a community's health problems, but, more importantly, we also discover a community's assets and strengths—the cultural capital needed to accomplish the goals of *Healthy People 2020.* This chapter offers a protocol for gathering, organizing, and interpreting information about the culture of a community.

CHAPTER 5 OBJECTIVES

■ Learn a systematic and comprehensive procedure for gathering and recording the environment, population, and social organization of a community.

■ Develop strategies for identifying a community's assets and strengths as well as its health problems.

■ Use comparison and contextual analysis to determine the impact of community culture on health and illness.

COMMUNITY CULTURE INQUIRY

The assessment and analysis of community culture uses a process of community assessment developed by Conrad Arensberg (1954, 1955, 1961) and his work with Solon Kimball (Arensberg & Kimball, 1965) to facilitate the integration of anthropology in community development and social services. It approaches the study of communities through assessment of three interrelated aspects of a community:

- Its physical environment

- Its population

- Its social organization

Contained within each of these components of community culture are subcomponents, which, when assessed, provide additional information with which to gain a greater understanding of a community.

This community culture inquiry is not intended to be exhaustive; rather, it provides a systematic and meaningful framework in which to organize community-culture information based on similar categories. The most important goal is not to complete every category and subcategory but to have a spirit of curiosity and discovery as the community is assessed in an orderly, systematic way and to manage the information so that it is most useful. The skills the community/public health nurse uses to collect information for the community cultural inquiry include:

- A review of databases to identify relevant statistics specific to this community.

- Communication with key informants, stakeholders, and others from the community, each of whom provides valuable insights regarding the community's assets and areas in need of improvement.

- Direct observation of the community and its people and resources, as well as virtual observation of relevant Internet resources, such as mapping tools and community-related websites.

■ Research in literature sources to illuminate understanding of similar communities and target populations and to identify evidence-based community programs that may prove valuable for the community being assessed. As data are obtained and analyzed, a meaningful picture of the community—its assets and strengths—is identified along with its dimensions of weakness.

This holistic examination of the community's culture uses strategies that are not unlike the ethnographic methods used by anthropologists when they enter a culture unknown to them. Although the strategies may be similar, the goals of the community/public health nurse and the ethnographic researcher are quite different: The researcher is interested in developing new knowledge that will help explain the relationship of human behavior to health and illness, but the goal of the community/public health nurse is to gain a comprehensive understanding of community culture to build a community's capacity for better health. The nurse assesses for cultural capital that can be deployed to mobilize community action as well as to identify features of the community that may at first appear to be unrelated to health but, in fact, are valuable community assets for constructing and implementing a culture-based, healthy community agenda.

THE PHYSICAL ENVIRONMENT OF A COMMUNITY

The physical environment and geographic location of a community include the space and the time it occupies. The *spatial aspect* of a community refers to its natural dimensions (e.g., hills, rivers, forests, or oceans) as well as its human-made environment (e.g., highways, buildings, bridges, and street plans). Together, these compose the *setting* (e.g., rural county, urban neighborhood, or coastal village) in which the target populations work and live (Eberhardt & Pamuk, 2004). In addition to space, the physical environment of a community occupies time. Communities have a history and a future that influence what can be accomplished in the present. They outlive individual members and successive generations, ranging from infants to seniors, and reflect an orderly progression of the population through days, seasons, and years. The community's history and future ambitions are just as much a part of community life as its rivers, roads, and buildings.

SPATIAL DIMENSIONS OF COMMUNITY LIFE

Communities occupy and use space and its contents in different ways and are shaped by it. For example, many of the original cities that grew in the northeastern United States were built around a waterfall to power the textile or paper mills on which their economies were based. The typical settlement pattern in such communities consisted of worker houses built on flat ground, while the owners and high-level managers lived in more elegant accommodations in the hills. Examples of this type of settlement can be found in communities throughout New England. Midwestern rural and agricultural communities, in comparison, were settled on farms and in family-dominated clusters of houses located in a more egalitarian manner, along roads leading to the town's "main street" commercial and service centers.

The spatial aspect of community life is a good place to initiate a culturally informed community assessment, because it does not necessitate extensive interviews or informal discussions with residents. Through direct observation, reference to maps, reviews of community and industry web pages, and drawings of community diagrams, much can be learned about a community, its assets and resources, and its potential and actual health problems. Most communities have fairly detailed maps that can be obtained from the Internet, local planning departments, or municipal or county offices. Popular mapping resources on the Internet that can be helpful include Google Earth, Google Maps, and SimplyMap.

A formal map is a good place to start; however, regardless of the availability of Internet mapping resources, driving around and walking through the community give the nurse a closer perspective on the major topographical features and social institutions.

POPULATION BOUNDARIES, SIZE, AND DISTRIBUTION

Suggested Activity

Do the following:

- Explore a community virtually using Internet mapping tools, such as Google Maps, Google Earth, and SimplyMap. Supplement the information by obtaining and reviewing a street map of the community.

- Tour the community (e.g., drive and/or walk it, always keeping safety in mind) and draw a map of the space, including natural and human-made topographical features and social organizations.

- Identify the physical boundaries of the community.

- Record the size of the community (e.g., in square miles).

Critical Thinking Questions: What additional discoveries have I made during this activity? What additional information would be helpful for me to include?

Community/public health nursing practice begins with knowing where nursing and healthcare services are to be provided. It is therefore necessary to start by identifying the physical boundaries and the size, expressed in square miles, of the geo-political territory to be served. Depending on the type of community, the size of its population, and the way in which people are distributed, it could be geographically small, such as a city block, or it could encompass several rural counties. The physical size of a community in square miles will strongly influence the amount of funding and resources available for community practice. Providing community/public health nursing services for a large population concentrated in a few city blocks is likely to be very different from, but equally as demanding as, providing services for a small population scattered over many square miles.

REGIONAL POSITION

Suggested Activity

Acquire a map that demonstrates the regional position of the community. Then do the following:

- Identify whether the community is a town, county, borough, village, or part of a municipality.

- Identify types of services that are available to community members. What resources are needed to access these services (e.g., transportation, membership, or insurance)?

- Identify where and how far community residents need to go to obtain various services.

- Describe commuting relationships between this community and other communities. What are the implications for daily living activities, such as work, kinship, and leisure?

- Determine the distance, in time and miles, to the nearest urban center.

- Read a local news source and speak to local community members to explore how the community relates to the geo-political units in which it is located.

Critical Thinking Questions: What additional discoveries have I made during this activity? What additional information would be helpful for me to include?

The regional position of a community indicates how it is situated in relation to other communities—whether it is a satellite to a larger city or other municipality or it is a center to which smaller communities are linked on a daily basis. The degree to which it is isolated from surrounding communities will influence the community's strengths and problems. For example, in a community that is remote, the community/public health nurse may need to mobilize lay community members to become health educators or emphasize self-help programs, such as first-aid readiness and health literacy. When trusting relationships with community members are cultivated, there can be many advantages to working in communities where kinship and neighbor networks provide meaningful social support and can be mobilized more easily.

The regional position of the community is significant, because many problems cannot be resolved merely at the local level. For example, people may live in community A but are getting sick where they work, in community B. These commuters who travel from the suburbs to the city and back to the suburbs may unknowingly be transmitting communicable diseases from one location to another.

In addition to work ties, strong social ties often exist between members of communities that are widely separated geographically. For example, many Puerto Rican families living in New York City send their children to Puerto Rico during summer vacations to stay with grandparents. It would be difficult to understand the culture of the specific neighborhoods in New York City without consideration of these families' ties in Puerto Rico. Similarly, it is not unusual for migrant farm workers in the Midwest to return to their home countries when the harvesting season is over to check on their relatives and, for some, to seek less-expensive healthcare.

GEO-PHYSICAL AND CLIMATE FACTORS

Suggested Activity

Do the following:

- Identify the natural features of the environment that serve as an organizing force in the district/community (e.g., rivers, mountains, plains, or coast).

- Identify the human-made features of the environment that serve as quasi-organic forces (e.g., superhighways, high-rise apartment complexes, industrial parks, bridges, tunnels, shopping malls, and sports arenas).

- Record the climate conditions of the area (e.g., precipitation, winds, and temperature range).

> Critical Thinking Questions: What additional discoveries have I made during this activity? What additional information would be helpful for me to include?

A community's geo-physical and climate factors, such as mountains, rivers, or coastline, may be organizing forces in community life. New construction sites are common features of the landscape on urban island settlements, such as Hong Kong, Singapore, and Manhattan, where older buildings are regularly being razed and replaced by newer, taller ones. In contrast, such cities as Los Angeles and Dallas sprawl indefinitely into their environments. Although some geo-physical and climate features, such as mudslides, floods, forest fires, and earthquakes, impose various threats to the health of a community, others provide opportunities for recreation and community gatherings. Human-made physical features, such as multilane highways, bridges, tunnels, and clusters of high-rise buildings or industrial parks, serve as semiorganic forms that affect the health of communities and human activity. For example, superhighways, uniting several communities, help centralize social and economic activities, expanding support for a healthy community agenda. At the same time, they may physically divide previously connected neighborhoods and contribute to potential health hazards, such as traffic accidents, air pollution, and harmful noise levels.

LAND USE

Suggested Activity

Describe how land in the community is designated for use (e.g., residential, recreational, commercial, industrial, agricultural, official, and spiritual or religious use). Describe the patterns of land use by the people in the community:

- Areas used by all members of the community
- Areas used by specific community members (e.g., old, young, women, and ethnic groups)

> ■ Areas used by organizations (e.g., local businesses, corporate enterprises, and government)
>
> Critical Thinking Questions: What additional discoveries have I made during this activity? What additional information would be helpful for me to include?

Communities create various kinds of boundaries. Some have settlement patterns with sections of the community designated for specific purposes, such as residential, commercial, industrial, governmental, spiritual, or recreational use. In other communities, residents sleep, eat, work, play, and worship within the range of a few blocks; there is no geographical separation of various community activities. The designation of different locations for different community functions generates patterns where community members live, work, congregate, and play. Areas used by local residents, government, and corporate interests may differ in community history and community engagement. Commercial centers, houses of worship, recreational centers, schools, or industrial complexes bring community members together for certain periods of the day or week, while their widely scattered homes take them in separate directions for the remainder of the time. It is important to identify areas where people congregate naturally to reach many residents at the same time. For example, in some communities, the most efficient way to reach larger numbers of adults might be through their places of employment, while in others it may be at religious services. These locations where people congregate naturally are part of a community's cultural capital and may be leveraged for health-promotion purposes.

Communities may be organized according to special characteristics of the residents, such as ethnicity or religion (e.g., Little Italy, an Amish community, or Chinatown), by economic class (e.g., the "ghettos"), or even by occupation, such as enclaves of artists and musicians or university faculty. Health disparities may be prevalent in subcultures within a community. In addition, many communities have been and continue to be characterized by segregation (Acevedo-Garcia, Lochner, Osypuk, & Subramanian, 2003), which was one of the principal reasons for the movement to desegregate school districts. Specific groups may informally designate a particular area of the community as their own "turf" and create boundaries that are not visible to the outsider but are well known and well respected by local residents.

A community has unspoken "rules" by which residents abide, and they govern where people go in a community. These rules have important implications for health planning and intervention. For example, a lead-screening program was held at a fast-food restaurant on a Saturday. A favorite gathering spot for young families on the weekend, the restaurant was considered an ideal site for reaching preschool-age children. In terms of the number of children screened, it was extremely successful; however, in terms of reaching the population most at risk, the program failed. No one had taken into consideration that the lower-income families with the highest-risk children who were most likely to have lead exposure would be unlikely to bring their children to a fast-food restaurant outside their own neighborhood. A better understanding of the use of space by people in the community and how different groups have different access to space could easily have averted the problem and saved the expense of an additional program.

HOUSING

Suggested Activity

Describe and/or create a "photo journal" documenting the following:

- Acquire pictures of the range of housing types in the community. What are the worst and the best housing conditions?

- Describe housing options available for lower-income community members.

- Map the types of housing on a street map.

- List the number of housing units by single family, multiple family, and high-rise apartment building. For example, do you observe group homes for people with disabilities, dormitories, assisted-living facilities, nursing homes, homeless shelters, and domestic-violence shelters?

- Describe the quality and types of structures. For example, do homes have broken or boarded windows? Are homes in disrepair, or are they well-maintained?

- Describe community members' access to community flower and vegetable gardens, open green spaces, lawns, parks, and recreational spaces.

- Identify types of housing materials. For example, are houses made of wood frame, cement, brick, thatch, mud, cardboard box, or tents? Do you observe asbestos use or lead-based chipped paint? Do houses have screens or open windows?

- Describe special housing features. For example, do homes use solar energy? Do houses in high-risk regions have radon-abatement systems? What other special features do you notice as you observe the various kinds of residences?

- Record the ages and conditions of housing.

- List utilities available in dwellings. For example, do they include water, lighting, cooking facilities, heating, air conditioning, and waste disposal?

Critical Thinking Questions: What additional discoveries have I made during this activity? What additional information would be helpful for me to include?

Housing plays an important role in providing a safe, healthy, comfortable, and aesthetically pleasing context for individual and family growth. In addition to providing shelter and protection from the elements, housing is directly related to the quality of family relationships and to the psychological and physical dimensions of health. The type of construction and the placement of housing units in relation to each other and to community gathering points influence the ways in which residents interact. For example, apartment buildings with a common courtyard, swimming pool, or laundry area may be more likely to foster more interaction among building residents than a high-rise, dormitory-like building where one rarely sees the person who lives in the apartment next door. Many cities, such as Chicago, have replaced high-rise dwellings with three-story, townhouse-type housing for this reason.

Access to a piece of land for gardens or recreation is another important feature of housing. Many innovative urban planners have transformed vacant lots into vegetable gardens, subdivided and tended by community members. In addition to solving the aesthetic and safety problems that accompany vacant lots, such gardens provide city residents with the opportunity to produce, preserve, and perhaps even sell fresh food. Such community gardens also can become a focal point for community activity, such as outdoor markets, and they can bring urban residents together and help improve access to fresh foods for some populations that may otherwise reside in food deserts.

Housing must be examined in relation to the characteristics of the people residing in the community. It may be very difficult for immigrants who were living in adobe, single-story homes with detached kitchens to adjust to the high-rise housing of urban centers. Housing units that were constructed for one group, such as young families, may not work as well for elders who require elevators, wheelchair ramps, and perhaps different kinds of lighting. Most modern housing is electricity-dependent and subject to energy crises in summer or winter months, creating a potentially serious problem for older adults. Finally, abandoned housing has generated a widespread community-safety problem, attracting gang members, illicit-drug users, and homeless urban squatters.

TRANSPORTATION

Suggested Activity

Do the following:

- Obtain transit maps of buses, subways, ferries, and waterways. Include a list of the costs of transportation.

- Map patterns of movement within and between residences, workplaces, commercial centers, healthcare centers, recreation centers, and schools.

- Outline major arteries, available routes, and public and private transportation options.

- Identify the dominant means of transportation observed. For example, list the use of private vehicles, public transportation, taxicabs, trains, bicycles, walking paths, skateboards, or other means of transportation.

- Describe the transportation links between the community and the nearest urban centers. How accessible are key health-related resources to the community's most vulnerable persons (e.g., persons who are elderly, disabled, in poverty, or homeless)?

- Identify the locations of sidewalks and their safety for residents in the community.

- List the methods of community-wide communications (e.g., texting alert systems, radio stations, and severe weather and emergency alerts) that serve the community.

- List the ways people receive news and information. Include newspapers, bulletins, television, the Internet and electronic resources popularly used in the community (e.g., smartphone apps, Facebook pages, Twitter, Instagram, and other forms of social media), and those that provide public health programs.

> ▪ Identify the accessibility of Internet connections and the presence and use of social media.
>
> ▪ Describe social marketing methods used, including social media resources as well as billboard advertising. What health topics are featured?
>
> Critical Thinking Questions: What additional discoveries have I made during this activity? What additional information would be helpful for me to include?

The designation of different zones for various community functions and events requires a transportation system to move people from one activity to another. In addition to knowing how land is used in the community, it also is necessary to understand the ways in which people use the network of roads, waterways, and other public transportation. This is especially important for the most vulnerable groups of people, who may have limited resources or abilities to reach health services.

> When a hospital in a large city decided to close its pediatric clinic, a nearby hospital began to plan for the influx of families it assumed would be drawn from the closed service. It was the closest hospital by distance; however, the journey required a transfer from one bus line to another. Most mothers found it more convenient to go to another clinic that was actually farther away but could be reached on one bus line, without the inconvenience of a transfer.

COMMUNICATION

The communication system is a critical capacity-building tool. Social media, cell phones and text messaging, radio, television, newspapers, and the Internet link individuals and groups within and outside the community for health education, disaster preparedness, and public participation in health planning and policy. Health editors of blogs, smartphone apps and popular Facebook pages, local newspapers, school principals, physical education teachers, school nurses, local television and radio health programs, religious leaders of local houses of worship, and church bulletins are examples of cultural capital that can be mobilized to disseminate information about health and to encourage the participation of community residents in health programs. Some nurses have launched newspaper columns, smartphone apps, Facebook pages, blogs, and television and radio programs to bring health information to the public. Internet services and social media are continuing to grow in their capacity for public communication, although the advantages of print media cannot be discounted: Health officials in a very ethnically diverse city found the most effective and efficient way to reach its multicultural population was through several well-read ethnic newspapers that each translated the information into the language of its readers. The community/public health nurse and community-partner health-promotion efforts will be most effective when you know the communication methods used by the various target populations within a community.

MENTAL MAPS

A famous cartoon depicts a New Yorker's perspective of the United States, which, looking west, includes first New Jersey and then the West Coast with nothing in between except Chicago; this is an example of a mental map. Persons living in Missouri, Montana, or Alabama are likely to have very different but perhaps equally distorted mental images of the United States. Community residents may also have a view of their surroundings that departs greatly from the actual geography. For several years, social scientists have used mental maps (including drawings by residents of their communities) to discover the interface of the psychological topography with the physical topography. In doing so, they have identified invisible peaks of psychological stress where residents are afraid to enter and valleys of safety where they feel comfortable and unafraid.

The names and nicknames applied to certain neighborhoods and sections of the community also tell much about how various neighborhoods are viewed. It is not unusual, for instance, for recently gentrified neighborhoods to have two names: one that is used by the residents who were born and grew up in the neighborhood and another that is used by the wealthier newcomers. This use of two names to describe the same place is telling: It may mirror social and economic differences between the two types of residents and suggest not only how various residents perceive themselves but also how they perceive others. It alerts us that there might be a need to use a different strategy for community action with each category of resident.

As with the "turf" aspects described earlier, sacred areas, areas of fear or safety, and other psychological features are superimposed on the physical features. Often, they are not obviously demarcated, so they may go unnoticed by the newcomer to the community. Sensitivity to mental maps is important, however, for understanding the perception people have of their environment and ensuring access to healthcare services for all populations in a community. Learning about the mental map of the community may be accomplished by reading about the community and its history, but most importantly by talking with various members who represent the diverse groups within the community.

Suggested Activity

Do the following:

- Record sections of the community distinguished by the residents themselves and the names or nicknames that are applied to them. When possible, speak with a cross-section of the community to gain different perspectives.

- Map the areas of the community that frequently are avoided or identified as unsafe.

- Map areas of the community that are designated as sacred or historical, such as ancient burial grounds and memorial parks.

Critical Thinking Questions: What additional discoveries have I made during this activity? What additional information would be helpful for me to include?

TEMPORAL DIMENSIONS OF COMMUNITY LIFE

Every community has daily, weekly, monthly, seasonal, semiannual, and annual cycles of activities that compose the cultural use of time. These temporal factors are especially important in community/public health nursing practice, because timeliness is often a critical factor for successful capacity building. If immunization programs are offered at a time when they are inaccessible to community residents, the participation rate will be low. Public health issues requiring legislative action are likely to get the most visibility and candidate support close to elections.

COMMUNITY HISTORY

Suggested Activity

Do the following:

- Determine the historical events that are important to the development and life of the community.

- Record the date and circumstances surrounding the settlement of the community.

- Describe patterns of population growth since the community was first settled, including waves of migration, immigration, and outmigration. Describe recent and current patterns of population growth or loss. What factors have contributed to these changes?

- What are examples of milestone events important to members of the community, including natural and human-made events? Examples include job growth or loss and economic changes; wars; major social events; community accomplishments; opening of new roads, railroads, or bridges; and disasters.

- Obtain a historical map of the community and designate the place and time of major physical alterations. If you do not have access to a historical map, ask longtime community members about major physical alterations.

■ Create a timeline of changes in community settlement patterns, such as a shift from downtown to suburban and then back to downtown.

■ Include major economic trends in the community on the timeline.

■ Include major political trends on the timeline.

Critical Thinking Questions: What additional discoveries have I made during this activity? What additional information would be helpful for me to include?

The community of today is largely a result of its history. Specific events and trends have worked to shape the place and its people. Knowledge of the history of the community is important for tracing and interpreting patterns of health problems over time and predicting those that will occur in the future. Understanding the local history is essential for strengthening a healthy community agenda by framing it in local traditions. Historical details of the community are not as important as a general knowledge of what has made the community what it is. A history may have already been written about the community that is available online or in the local library, either because the area has a particularly interesting history or because it was done as part of a community event or celebration. If no recorded history is available, explore other sources, such as interviews with older or longtime residents, newspaper series, public records, census reports, school records, directories, deeds and old maps, and church records.

CYCLICAL POPULATION MOVEMENT

To plan and implement public health action, it is very important to know the daily, weekly, seasonal, semiannual, and annual changes in the population. The movement of people from one place to another generally takes place with a degree of regularity and needs to be included in the community assessment to ensure the health and safety of community residents. For example, to ensure the safety of children coming and going to school, it is necessary to know when automobile traffic is heaviest and when children could be more likely to encounter risks to their safety.

Suggested Activity

Do the following:

- On daily and weekly schedules, identify routine community activities.
- On an annual calendar, record community events that take place each year.
- Identify seasonal changes in the community. What effects do seasonal changes have on the culture of the community?
- Record how community use of time varies with various segments of the population.

Critical Thinking Questions: What additional discoveries have I made during this activity? What additional information would be helpful for me to include?

Seasonal changes in the population often include major shifts in population, such as tourists and college-student workers who expand the population in the summer months on Cape Cod or double the population of Amherst, Massachusetts, from September to May. These seasonal fluctuations in population size have profound public health implications. The tourists who populate the New England ocean-resort towns and "snowbird" migrations of retired adults to Florida in the winter months present resource challenges for creating safe environments that range from water rescue to sanitation to restaurant inspection to traffic safety.

ECONOMIC CYCLES

This category of the community inventory includes temporal variations in the local economic structure, including cyclical variations in productivity, employment, occupation, income, and expenditures. The influence of seasonal variation in the local economy on health and healthcare is apparent in agricultural communities. In communities where agricultural sugar cane production is the main economic activity, for example, hundreds of workers are employed during a 6-month

Suggested Activity

Do the following:

- Record weekly, monthly, and seasonal work patterns, such as regular periods of unemployment, cycles of productivity, and seasonal occupational changes.

- Record periodic changes in income and expenditures. Ask a community member and a local business owner how the community is affected by population shifts.

Critical Thinking Questions: What additional discoveries have I made during this activity? What additional information would be helpful for me to include?

period in the field to cut the cane and in the factory to process it into sugar. During this time, cash is in the greatest circulation, and people have the resources to pay off their debts and make new purchases. It is also the time when utilization of healthcare services increases dramatically, reflecting that people are often taking care of problems that have been deferred during the leaner months. Additionally, seasonal work patterns and industries, such as agriculture and construction, have high rates of traumatic deaths (*Healthy People 2020*), requiring public health safety intervention.

PSYCHOLOGICAL CYCLES

Communities have periodic cycles when either psychological elevation or depression is generalized throughout the population. In most American communities, holidays and other times of ceremonial activity are seen as periods of high levels of anticipation and enthusiasm, with opportunities to be with family and to renew old friendships. These are also the time periods with the greatest incidence of suicide. Often, euphoric seasons are followed by dysphoric periods when the excitement of the holidays is over, work has resumed, bills must be paid, and weather keeps people indoors and isolated from friends and recreational activity.

The first warm days then bring a return of euphoria, with the anticipation of spring and summer and the resumption of social interaction and physical activity.

Suggested Activity

Chart on a 12-month calendar the psychological cycles of the community:

- When does the community experience periods of euphoria and dysphoria (e.g., memories and pride during football seasons; memories of sorrow from a community tragedy, such as a tornado, flood, or violent event)?

- Festivities and holidays: Are there community activities, such as parades and festivals, that take place during the year that commemorate local or national holidays or special events? What are the themes with a special identity that are important to some of or all the community members?

- Chart leisure and recreation periods in the community. Are there days of the week or seasons of the year typically used to relax, enjoy recreation, or vacation?

- Identify periods of widespread melancholy. What are the possible contextual and historical reasons for this occurrence?

Critical Thinking Questions: What additional discoveries have I made during this activity? What additional information would be helpful for me to include?

Student health centers report similar patterns. Each semester begins with the excitement of new classes and new friends. Then as the semester wears on, students are faced with assignments, tests, and papers to be completed, and a fairly predictable midterm dysphoria sets in. At that point, it is common to hear students say they cannot wait for the semester to be over and even express doubt as to whether they will be able to complete their course of study. During these periods of stress, absenteeism is most likely to occur, comparatively minor complaints take on an enhanced significance, and visits to health services increase. At the same time, faculty members feel equally stressed—perhaps in response to students—creating a system-wide emotional decline. In comparison, during periods of euphoria, it is not uncommon to hear students say, "I don't have time to get sick; I'm getting ready to go home for the holidays," or, "I'm not going to miss homecoming just because I have the flu." During these periods, complaints are minimized, and health-service utilization decreases.

CYCLICAL CRISES

Suggested Activity

Do the following:

- Chart recurring crises on an annual calendar/schedule, and determine whether these crises are experienced by some or most of the community members.

- List the sporadic crises that have occurred over the past 20 years. How well did the community cope with the crises? What factors contributed to effective or ineffective coping? How long did it take for community members to regain a sense of normalcy following a crisis?

Critical Thinking Questions: What additional discoveries have I made during this activity? What additional information would be helpful for me to include?

Practically all communities have crises that recur on a fairly predictable schedule. Spring flooding, annual flu epidemics, hurricane season, and winter fires are common examples of critical events that take place more or less regularly. According to *Healthy People 2020*, drowning, the second-leading cause of injury-related death in children and adolescents, is a seasonal event. Because seasonal events are relatively predictable, public health measures can be instituted to attempt to either prevent such events or minimize the damage that will accompany them. Some communities may experience an unexpected crisis of major proportion as a result of nature or a human-made disaster. Examples of natural crises include the effects of an F5 tornado that destroys a whole community; a major hurricane, such as Hurricane Katrina; or an out-of-control wildfire that rapidly burns many homes. Human-caused crises can create widespread emotional trauma, perhaps due to ethnic discord, gun violence, or the betrayal of trust of a public figure who turns out to be an embezzler or sexual abuser.

> Nurse midwives practicing in a remote and mountainous community reported bringing pregnant women across the river each year before the rainy season, when the normally shallow and easily fordable river began to swell. This is an example of anticipating problems and finding ways to ameliorate them or soften their impact.
>
> Following the unexpected shooting of a beloved public school teacher by a former student who became violent, the community deeply mourned the loss of the teacher. The community also mourned the imprisonment of the former student, who was once an endearing young person but developed a mental illness that went untreated due to barriers to care and lack of understanding about mental illness. The community deeply mourned this dual tragedy for many years following the event. A positive outcome was that gradually the community's conversations about the lack of mental-health services improved awareness and increased resources directed toward their development.

Community action can involve presenting a prevention program on summer safety, including water safety and first aid, at the end of the school year, which could reduce the number of events over the summer and equip children to provide assistance. Hurricanes, tornados, forest fires, seasonal floods, and other seasonal disasters require an educated citizenry who knows where to go and what to do to help others minimize the impact of a disaster.

In addition to the seasonal crises, other disasters have the potential to occur. Fires, tornadoes, tsunamis, earthquakes, major epidemics, mining disasters, nuclear disasters, and terrorist attacks all require preparation. The goal is to develop and maintain the community's capacity for readiness to reduce the impact of such an event by having a community plan in place. In a healthy community, the potential for such crises is identified, and a plan is in place for an interprofessional team that includes health- and human-service professionals, such as sanitation and safety engineers, police, communications networks, and rescue teams. In a healthy community, such problems as lack of health services or gun violence are identified, and culturally informed community action is mobilized.

THE POPULATION OF A COMMUNITY

An examination of a community's culture must include a review of the main reason a community exists: the people who live and work in the community. The number of people in a community and their attributes influence a community's ability to create a healthy future. The population can be examined as a whole, in terms of its size, growth, and distribution. It also can be examined in terms of the bio-cultural and socioeconomic characteristics of its members. These characteristics tell us much about the kinds of public health problems that can be anticipated; they also provide information about the strengths and assets of the population for facilitating a healthy community agenda. As you learned from studying communities, they experience environmental changes. This is also true of their populations. For example, a population's demographic profile may change, with a larger percentage of the population being age 65 and older. Additionally, depending on how it is defined, a population may include residents who spend only part of the year or part of the week in the community, or even those who come there every day for work or school but return to another community at night.

POPULATION SIZE, DENSITY, AND DISTRIBUTION

An understanding of the population begins with knowing not only how many people reside in the community but also how they are distributed. *Rural localities,* defined as communities with fewer than 2,500 residents, compose 25% of the American population. Some health-related needs are unique to rural conditions and lifestyles, and the Affordable Care Act is working to address them through the expansion of rural-community health center services. At the same time, we know that many urban neighborhoods also have unique public health issues, ranging from lack of affordable housing, street-safety problems, and gang violence to poor nutritional resources and food deserts due to an absence of grocery stores and fresh produce.

Suggested Activity

Do the following:

- Record the size of the population of the community.

- Identify weekly changes in the population. Do the numbers and characteristics of people in the community vary throughout the week?

- Identify seasonal changes in the population. Do the numbers and characteristics of people in the community vary by season?

- Describe the density of the population (that is, the number of people per square mile).

- Map the distribution of the population between urban and rural areas.

- Describe population changes and factors leading to those changes over the last 20 years. For example, consider economic changes, disasters, development of major businesses, and migration patterns. If migrating populations have recently entered the community, where are these people migrating from, and how is the community responding to their migration?

Critical Thinking Questions: What additional discoveries have I made during this activity? What additional information would be helpful for me to include?

Depending on the size of the community, it may contain urban and rural sections and areas of high and low population density. In addition to current size and density, changes in the population create new public health concerns. This begins with an accounting of population trends over the past several years, including patterns of migration—to *and* from the community—movement of immigrants and refugees, and natural increases or decreases in size, determined by birth and death rates. These population shifts can have a substantial impact on community resources and the healthcare system.

TEMPORARY SUBPOPULATIONS

Suggested Activity

Do the following:

- Identify the people who enter the community on a daily basis but do not live there.
- Identify the people who stay in the community on a weekly basis.
- Record the seasonal subpopulations residing in the community. Describe how many people are in the community during each season:
    - Tourists
    - Military personnel
    - Seasonal workers
    - Students

Critical Thinking Questions: What additional discoveries have I made during this activity? What additional information would be helpful for me to include?

Some communities include special groups, such as military personnel, summer residents, students, migrant workers, or other groups who may *reside* in the community but are not *of* the community. In some instances, such groups may contribute to the economy of the community and bring positive attributes that enhance the cultural capital of the community. On the other hand, they may strain community resources, compromising the community's capacity for health. In any case, the presence of these groups must be accounted for to ensure the future health of the community. This includes identifying their numbers, major characteristics, roles within the community, strengths, prevailing health risks and problems, and the resources they can offer to build the community's capacity for health.

BIOLOGICAL COMPOSITION: AGE AND SEX

Suggested Activity

Do the following:

- Record the median age of the population.
- List the percentages of the population who are in the following age ranges: 0 to 5, 6 to 14, 15 to 19, 20 to 34, 35 to 49, 50 to 64, 65 and over, as well as the older population subgroupings of 65 to 74, 75 to 84, and 85 and over.
- Compute the dependency ratio of the population.
- Identify the sex composition of the population. How many people identify as male, female, homosexual, bisexual, transgender, or other?
- Identify the sex ratio of the population based on the sex composition.
- Compute the age/sex quotient of the population based on the sex composition.

Critical Thinking Questions: What additional discoveries have I made during this activity? What additional information would be helpful for me to include?

When providing direct care to individual patients, it is necessary to know their biological characteristics to make accurate nursing diagnoses and formulate appropriate care plans. The same principle holds true when providing care to an entire community. The age and sex distribution of a population tells us much about the kinds of health concerns that residents of the community are likely to experience now and in the future, as well as their impact on the health of the community. Age and sex are, perhaps, the most fundamental of the biological characteristics, because so many community health problems are linked to gender and stage of development. For example, the aging of populations and reduction in communicable diseases throughout the United States have mandated a shift in a major emphasis from infectious disease and child health to management of chronic illness and the needs of elder community residents.

In statistical compilations, the *age of a population* is presented as the percentage of the population that falls into prescribed categories. The utility of age categories, however, depends on the community. For example, if a setting has a large proportion of older adult citizens, the "over 65" group might be subdivided into "young elders," ages 65 to 74; "mid-elders," ages 75 to 84; and "frail elders," ages 85 and over. At the same time, two of the adult categories might be collapsed into one large group from ages 35 to 64, simply because the community does not have large numbers of individuals in those particular age groups. In other words, the categories should be refined in a way that reflects and is most useful for the particular community being evaluated.

The proportion of the population that is typically not in the labor force is considered to be more likely economically and socially dependent on the rest of the population and is therefore computed as the *dependency ratio*. The dependency ratio is the number of people ages 0 to 14 plus the number of people ages 65 and older, divided by the number of people ages 15 to 64. It also is the proportion of the population that is likely to require the most health resources. It is therefore a significant figure for public health considerations.

Men, women, and transgendered people differ in the kinds of health problems they experience and the manner and frequency with which they use health services. Acknowledging that some sex-specific health problems are biologically based, *Healthy People 2020* highlights gender as one of the five categories in which health disparities must be addressed, yet it emphasizes that the longer life expectancy in females cannot be attributed solely to biological factors (National Center for Health Statistics, 2012). The *sex ratio* of a community helps us understand and predict prevailing health concerns and the need for resources. As the sex that bears children and generally lives longer, it is not surprising that women use more health services than men do. Furthermore, health problems that were once attributable primarily to the male population, such as cardiovascular disease, now are emerging with increasing frequency among females. A high sex ratio—that is, a predominance of either males or females—signals a need to review community services for men, women, and children.

Once the age and sex composition of the community has been determined, it is useful to cross-tabulate these two factors to determine the sex ratio in each age category. This greater refinement of age and sex data permits even more predictability as each age group moves to the next developmental stage. For example, it is usually assumed that the ages-65-and-older category is predominantly female, but a closer investigation of the community may reveal that military service and migration have left particular communities lacking in males in one age group but increasing in proportion in another. For several years, the older adult population in Chinese communities in many U.S. cities was predominantly male, reflecting the wave of Chinese immigrant men who came to the United States in the first half of the 20th century as laborers. As each age group moves through its next developmental sequence, its sex composition will have an impact on the health of the community and the necessary health services.

ETHNIC AND RACIAL GROUPS

Race and ethnicity constitute another of the factors highlighted by *Healthy People 2020* that are linked to health disparities in this country. According to the U.S. Census Bureau, approximately 36.3% of the U.S. population belongs to a racial- or ethnic-minority population (U.S. Census Bureau, 2008b). Ethnicity and race are two distinct categories that often are misapplied (Drevdahl, Phillips, & Taylor, 2006; Phillips & Drevdahl, 2003; Wolf, 1994). *Ethnicity* is the complex of traits that identify a group of people based on such characteristics as common ancestry, language, and/or religion. *Race*, on the other hand, is a more controversial concept. Although we commonly think of race as a biological attribute based on a person's phenotype and genotype, contemporary social science conceptualizes race as a socially constructed category. In the United States, for example, a person whose appearance (or phenotype) is "White" is often considered "Black" if his mother happens to be African American. "Hispanic" is a common racial category on health and census surveys, implying, incorrectly, that people of Spanish origin are a separate racial group from White or Black.

Suggested Activity

Do the following:

- List the various ethnic/racial groups found in the community.
- Calculate each ethnic/racial group's percentage of the total population.
- Record the percentage of the population that identifies itself as multiracial.
- Determine the homogeneity or diversity of the various racial and ethnic groups.

Critical Thinking Questions: What additional discoveries have I made during this activity? What additional information would be helpful for me to include?

Neither race nor ethnicity can be determined from an individual's phenotype or genotype. But because census reports and health surveys often use categories that label people as White, Black, or Hispanic, it is important to have a basic understanding of race. With the geographical clustering of populations and a resultant common gene pool, it is not unusual for specific health problems to have genetic origins and thus appear with greater frequency in some groups than in others. It is well known, for example, that sickle-cell anemia is found more often in African American and Caribbean American populations, Tay-Sachs disease in some Jewish groups, skin cancer in those of northern European ancestry, and diabetes in American Indian groups. Certain groups also have inherited resistance to specific diseases. Cancer rates, for instance, are comparatively low in American Indian populations. Thus, at the community level, race and ethnicity can inform the identification of risk for problems likely to require public health action, such as screening and health education.

Many health problems correlated with particular ethnic groups are not caused by an inherited predisposition but rather from the social position, socioeconomic status, or conditions of employment of particular groups or subgroups. The combination of biological and social factors can result in variable health status. For example, the higher rate of hypertension in some African American and other groups has been related to the stress associated with a lifetime of discrimination (Dressler, 2004). Race and ethnicity have a profound influence on the health and sustainability of communities. They can be the source of community conflict, isolation, uneven distribution of resources, poor health, and, ultimately, health disparities. On the other hand, diversity can richly enhance cultural capital and be a source of strength in mobilizing and uniting communities.

Prejudice and discrimination have not been confined to groups of color, as the histories of the Irish and of the Eastern European Jews in 19th- and early-20th-century America attest. In cases where discrimination has been legally sanctioned, such as with African-American populations until the 1950s, the quality and quantity of prejudice have been particularly deplorable. For example, well into the 20th century, laws prohibited African Americans from patronizing many restaurants, hotels, healthcare facilities, and educational institutions. The unique circumstances of African-American populations must be acknowledged to appreciate the vast differences in opportunity that have characterized various ethnic and racial groups over time (Carlson & Chamberlain, 2004).

Suggested Activity

On the *Healthy People 2020* home page, compare the leading cause of death among the different ethnic and racial populations.

OCCUPATION, INCOME, AND EDUCATION LEVEL

Suggested Activity

Do the following:

- Record the per capita income in the community.
- Record the mean and median family income and household income.
- Record the percentage of the population with an income below the poverty level.
- Record the percentage of school-age children receiving "free and reduced lunch" services.
- Record the percentage of the population receiving public assistance.
- Record the unemployment rate by age and sex.
- Identify the percentage of females in the workforce.
- List the major occupational categories of the population—for example, professionals, technical workers, managers, officials, proprietors, artisans, operatives, farmers, laborers, and domestic workers. Which occupations are considered "high risk"?
- Evaluate the mean and median income in relation to the cost of living. Ask local community members what they know about income sufficiency and the cost of living.
- Determine the percentage of the population over age 25 that has completed high school.
- Determine the percentage of the population over age 25 that has completed college.

Critical Thinking Questions: What additional discoveries have I made during this activity? What additional information would be helpful for me to include?

Income, occupation, and education influence many aspects of health and health-care. There is no question that populations with high rates of unemployment, poverty, and public assistance will experience more public health problems (Rodwin & Neuberg, 2005; Szwarcwald, da Mota, Damacena, & Pereira, 2011; Webb, Simpson, & Hairston, 2011). Generally, the problems in poorer communities are more complex, because the resources to resolve them are less accessible. According to the Secretary's Advisory Committee on National Health Promotion and Disease Prevention Objectives for 2020, inequality in income is highlighted as a key social and physical environmental-health determinant underlying health disparities (*Healthy People 2020*).

Interpreting the impact of occupation and income requires evaluating indicators, such as average income per household, within the local economic context. For example, an average family income of $50,000 per year may be more than sufficient to meet the household needs of families living in some rural areas of the United States but totally inadequate for a similar family residing in Southern California or Boston, Massachusetts. Differences in economic profile are associated with other differences, such as age distribution or ethnicity. Evaluating the income level of a population must be done in relation to the cost of living within the same region.

In addition to the income level, the occupational composition of the population affects the health of a community. For example, mining and textile manufacturing pose high public health risks for respiratory problems. The proportion of adult females in the workforce signals the need to determine the effects of employment and occupation on women's health, including fertility. It also raises the question of whether there is a sufficient number of high-quality day care centers for the young children of working mothers.

Finally, mothers' education levels are a universal predictor of child health and development worldwide. Because a large component of public health intervention is educational, the educational and health-literacy statuses of women in the community are important indicators. Education, similar to income, requires evaluation in relation to the context. In some communities, a high-school education is meaningful and will be the standard even for the community's most prominent citizens. In other communities, it may represent the most minimal preparation.

RESIDENTIAL AND HOUSEHOLD CHARACTERISTICS

Suggested Activity

Do the following:

- Record the percentage of the population over age 16 that is currently single, married, divorced, and widowed.

- Determine the number of family units in the community.

- Determine the average population per household.

- Record the percentage of single-person households in the community.

- Record the number of owner-occupied households.

- Record the number of tenant-occupied households.

- Record the percentage of the population living in substandard housing.

- Record shelters or temporary housing available for vulnerable groups of people, such as homeless people, domestic-violence victims, runaway youth, and people with disabilities. Describe the quality of housing available.

- Record the percentage of community members that reside in Section 8 (low-income) housing. Is this type of housing available in a single region of the community, or is it scattered throughout the community?

Critical Thinking Questions: What additional discoveries have I made during this activity? What additional information would be helpful for me to include?

Different kinds of household configurations distinguish neighborhoods and communities. The prevailing domestic units may consist of young singles or old singles, single parents and their children, grandparents and grandchildren, or any number of combinations, as well as the conventional nuclear family. Because the household generally is the unit of personal healthcare, it is important to know how many households are in the district. A population of 3,000 divided into 500 households will create very different public health considerations than a population of 3,000 divided into 1,500 households. One-person households may present special public health challenges, especially if the person is disabled or in the senior-citizen age group.

Because most people spend one- to two-thirds of their lives at home, housing has a profound influence on the health of the population, including the growth and development of children and the functioning of families. Households considered crowded or substandard in one community may be acceptable in another community. The number of owner-occupied homes as opposed to renter-occupied homes often is used to indicate the stability and investment of residents in making their community a safe and attractive place to live. In some communities, however, renters are highly invested in their neighborhoods—emotionally and economically—and are as vigilant as homeowners are about maintaining the quality of their buildings and their community.

THE SOCIAL ORGANIZATION OF A COMMUNITY

In *Healthy People 2020*, one of the overarching goals includes creating social and physical environments that promote good health for all groups. Social environments are linked to health-related quality of life and life satisfaction. According to the U.S. Department of Health and Human Services in *Healthy People 2010*:

> The social environment has a profound effect on individual health, as well as on the health of the larger community, and is unique because of cultural customs; language; and personal, religious or spiritual beliefs. (p. 19)

The three lenses through which we will describe and analyze the social relationships and interactions that compose the community's culture are as follows:

- Community institutions

- Horizontal stratification of the community

- Vertical segmentation of the community

COMMUNITY INSTITUTIONS

Institutions are standardized patterns of social behavior typified by a regular cycle of activities, specific groupings and personnel, and an accompanying set of rules and ideology. The presence and ongoing functioning of institutions give a community its character and its sense of stability. When an activity or a social behavior is institutionalized, it is no longer dependent on a specific person or persons to make it happen. Rather, it has taken on a life of its own. The institution of marriage is a good example. It is not something each individual invents as he or she reaches adulthood, for it is an established social pattern. And although each person has a choice of whether to partake in the institution of marriage, it is nonetheless clearly established as a normative expectation of adult life for many in our society. Marriage has a set of rules, formal and informal, that govern its performance. Formal rules relate, for example, to whom people can marry, the age at which a person can become married without parental consent, and who can officiate at a marriage. Less formal rules, on the other hand, might govern the appropriate age difference between marriage partners or who may be invited to a wedding.

Just because something is institutionalized does not mean it is incapable of change. It simply means change will require some kinds of societal reorganization. Using the same example, it is easy to see that the institution of marriage has undergone remarkable changes within the past 30 years. These changes include the following:

- The age at which many people are choosing to marry

- The ease with which a divorce is obtained

- The roles each of the partners assumes

- The number of times people are married

- The number of unmarried couples who live together

- The number of same-sex couples who live together or marry

Moreover, new institutions always are developing to meet societal needs that currently are not being addressed by existing institutions. The changing pattern of marriage in our society has created a need for standardized ways of dealing with divorce and the custody of children. Because divorce was less common in the past, the activities and rules surrounding becoming unmarried were not standardized, and each couple was left to work out a solution in its own way and on its own terms.

The community inquiry related to community institutions does not attempt to cover all aspects of culture or all the institutions that constitute a community's culture; rather, it explores the major categories of institutions that one is likely to find in almost all communities. They also are the most useful categories for guiding public health practice. They include economic, government, domestic, religion, education, and recreational and voluntary institutions. Depending on the community, different institutions assume different levels of significance, and institutions not included in the list may be more important to your assessment. *The critical factor is not a detailed account of every institution but the ability to identify institutions and understand how they are linked to the health of the community.* Health-related institutions have been omitted, intentionally, from this section, because they are discussed in detail in Chapter 6, "Determining the Health of Your Community," which focuses exclusively on health, the healthcare infrastructure, and institutional health organizations.

Economic Forces

Like all institutions, the economy of a community can be viewed as cultural capital and as cultural liability. Economic leaders can be powerful allies in making communities healthy places in which to work, raise families, live in quality housing, receive an education, and grow old comfortably. At the same time, the health of a community may be endangered by an economy dominated by greed and grounded in the exploitation of specific populations, the creation of social and health disparities, or the degradation of the environment and natural resources. *The degree to which economic opportunity, such as employment and financing, is available to all sectors of the population is an indication of the economic health of the community.*

Suggested Activity

Do the following:

- Describe the major economic base of the community—for example, manufacturing, industrial, wholesale, retail, resort, education, health, government center, commercial center, or diversified.
- Describe the relationship between employers and employees or workers and management.
- List the major employers in the community.
- Describe the role of workers' associations, such as unions.
- Chronicle the changes in the economy over the last 10 years.
- Summarize the effects these economic changes have had on the community.
- Describe the health and safety factors associated with local industry.

Critical Thinking Questions: What additional discoveries have I made during this activity? What additional information would be helpful for me to include?

Understanding the economy that fuels community life and the changes that have taken place over the years permits the most fundamental understanding of current and future health problems. In a healthy community, some resources are reinvested into the well-being of community members. In contrast, potentially dangerous ecological changes, environmental hazards, and/or the physical, psychological, and social problems associated with low wages or unemployment (Worthman & Kohrt, 2005) or job loss (Burgard, Brand, & House, 2007; Grunberg, Moore, Greenberg, & Sikora, 2008; Sikora, Moore, Greenberg, & Grunberg, 2008) can be caused by questionable economic values. These problems pose significant threats to the health and well-being of community members. An assessment of health and safety factors of the local economy involves two components:

- Economic impact on the environment, including air, noise, water, and food pollution

■ Economic direct influence on the health of citizens, including the conditions of employment, income, financial stress, and socioeconomic dislocations

In some communities, it is relatively easy to describe the local economy and its influence on community health, particularly if it has a single economic base—for example, a farming village, a tourist resort, or a manufacturing facility. In others, however, it may take several months or even years to reveal the true economic basis of a community. Many immigrant populations support their communities of origin with monthly remittances from relatives who have migrated to the United States. Similarly, communities may have an "underground" economy based on such activities as the sale of illicit drugs (Dreher, 1982b). In fact, the economic significance of such activities underlies much of the failure to reduce drug abuse in inner cities.

Government, Politics, and Law-Enforcement Issues

Government is the official structure, set of activities, and officials entrusted with the authority to make decisions on behalf of the community and to create and enforce the laws and policies that administer the community. *Politics* is a system of social relations in which access to and exercise of power are played out through *law enforcement* and in which *power* is defined most elementally as the ability to influence. Although politics exists at every level of human organization, people feel the effects most keenly at the local level of government. This is where governmental decisions enter the lives of citizens on a daily basis, such as the schools their children attend, the roads on which they drive, the police protection they receive, how their property is zoned, how waste is removed and sanitized, and the taxes they pay. A community culture inquiry must include the identity of local public officials, how they were vested with authority (elected, appointed, or inherited), and how they vote on issues of health and welfare. This is essential information for explaining current health issues, understanding current public health priorities and programs, and mobilizing the community for future health action. Political parties may or may not be represented at the most local level, and it is not uncommon to have two or three independent candidates running for office, each with his or her own individual agenda and constituency. On the other hand, many communities have a dominant political-party affiliation that party leaders acknowledge through governmental assistance in return for community-wide support.

Suggested Activity

Do the following:

- Describe the formal structure of the local government.

- Identify local sources of public revenue (property and sales taxes).

- Describe the election process.

- List the elected representatives for the community and their party affiliations.

- Summarize the political-party representation in the community, including recent trends.

- Describe the law-enforcement organization for the district.

- Describe the penal system.

- Describe community members' perceptions of how accessible and responsive local representatives are to community members.

- Describe community members' perceptions of the sufficiency of the law-enforcement and penal systems in the community.

- List any current or recent political controversies in the community. Are any community health implications associated with these controversies?

- Summarize the local government's health department and officials responsible for overseeing the health of the community (e.g., list the main programs of the local health department).

- Specify the local government's budget for health.

- Specify the voting records of elected officials on health issues.

Critical Thinking Questions: What additional discoveries have I made during this activity? What additional information would be helpful for me to include?

The *tax structure* is the place in which economic institutions and political institutions come together. The concern of citizens over an increasing tax burden created by government initiatives—no matter how wholesome for the public they may be—is very real and can be a major deterrent in planning and implementing a healthy community agenda. The scattering of nuclear power plants throughout the northeast corridor of the United States in previous decades, for example, provided tax relief as well as employment opportunities for the citizens of small towns. Although this trend generated some local resistance—centered mainly on health and safety hazards for future generations—the short-term tax-reduction advantages to citizens were difficult to counter.

Domestic Issues

The terms *household* and *family* often are used synonymously, generally because in American society, they often refer to the same group of people. Family, however, refers to those related by kinship ties, whether by blood, adoption, marriage, or convention; and household refers to those who share a living space. Although these are grossly oversimplified definitions, it is easy to see that depending on how family is defined, it is possible to have households composed of more than one family and families comprising more than one household. Communities differ greatly in the ways their populations are organized into families and households. Some are divided into single-household units, occupied by nuclear families consisting of a mother and a father or a same-sex couple and their unmarried children. Others are much more complex and contain a variety of domestic arrangements. Extended families may occupy several households located in proximity, with extensive and routine visiting among them. In migrant-worker and refugee communities, it is not uncommon to have several unrelated individuals and families occupying the same household.

The household is just as important as the family. Households generally are composed of people who eat and sleep in the same dwelling and who are in routine (usually daily) contact. It is common for household members to have mutual care-giving functions, although it is not at all unusual for these functions to be shared by family members and others who are not part of the household. Because the household often is the unit of personal healthcare, trends in household structure and the implications for the health of the public are important to monitor. In some communities, it is not uncommon for multiple individuals who are unknown to each other to rent separate bedrooms but share the rest of the house. This type of household may entail no familial or close relationship, but the space and facilities are shared, and the residents live in close contact. This kind of housing arrangement can be seen in communities with a shortage of housing or where the cost of renting one's own space is prohibitive.

Suggested Activity

Do the following:

- Describe the variation in domestic composition of households.

- Report the percentage of single-parent households.

- Determine the average number of children per household.

- Report the percentage of unmarried heterosexual couples living together.

- Report the percentage of unmarried same-sex couples living together.

- Ascertain the expected roles of family members—for example, mother/father, husband/wife, child/parent, and child/grandparent. Identify distinctions that exist in same-sex couple households.

- Describe the norms and rules governing courtship and marriage.

- Determine the legal age for marriage without parental consent for heterosexual and same-sex couples.

- Find out the average age at which people are first married.

- Report the rates of divorce, separation, and annulment.

Critical Thinking Questions: What additional discoveries have I made during this activity? What additional information would be helpful for me to include?

The norms governing family, marital, and domestic life underpin some of our most ingrained institutions and often differ widely from culture to culture. It is imperative to set aside our own values regarding domestic life and not criticize how families are organized in households in other communities. For example, rather than supposing that the children of divorced parents are victims of a broken family, we could reframe them as children who have the benefit of belonging to two households with loving and protective parents. Moreover, in situations where there is only one parent, unofficial or "adopted" mothers and fathers often emerge from among friends, relatives, and neighbors to create a more healthful psychological environment than that which existed when the biological parents occupied the same household.

Another kind of family structure that has emerged over the past two decades is that of same-sex couples, including those who have married or publicly declared their commitment and share a residence, sometimes also raising children. Most recently, the Supreme Court has declared the right of same-sex couples to marry, although it continues to be controversial in some states and communities. Because the level of social acceptance of a gay/lesbian sexual orientation has been uneven, *Healthy People 2010* set forth sexual identity and orientation as a topic in which health disparities occurred. In *Healthy People 2020*, lesbian, gay, transgender, and bisexual health has been added as a new topic area.

For gay men, health issues include HIV/AIDS, substance abuse, depression, and suicide, while for lesbian women, some evidence points to higher rates of smoking, alcohol abuse, obesity, and stress. For both groups, personal safety and mental health are critically important issues (*Healthy People 2020*). The CDC State of Aging and Health in America report (2013, p. iii) has prioritized the need to address lesbian, gay, bisexual, and transgender (LGBT) aging and health issues.

The social conventions pertaining to the sequence of courting, living together, marrying, and having children differ greatly from society to society. Some couples choose to not marry yet live as committed partners, often due to economic considerations. For those who marry, marriage may be arranged without a period of courtship, and pregnancy may occur without marriage. In some cultures, it is common to attend a marriage ceremony in which all the children (and sometimes the grandchildren) of the couple are members of the wedding party. Traditions that may appear exotic to the outsider are supported in their communities (Dreher & Hudgins, 2010; McElroy & Townsend, 2004).

Religion

Suggested Activity

Do the following:

- List, by religious affiliation, the churches, temples, mosques, and other places of worship attended by residents in the community, and locate them on the map.

- Determine the size and average attendance and days and times of the week that each congregation participates in religious activities.

- Identify whether the congregations have websites and which elements of the groups and/or worship centers could potentially be leveraged for the healthy community agenda and/or community action.

- Identify which religious groups are increasing in membership and which are decreasing.

- List the names of the clergy of the various churches and/or worship centers.

- Describe the role each religious facility plays in the healthcare of the community (e.g., does it have a parish or faith-community nurse?).

- Identify the religious groups that have taken leadership positions for neighborhood or community health activities.

- Identify minority religious groups in the community.

- Identify agnostic/atheist groups in the community.

- Describe religious expression observed in the community (e.g., Crosses, Star of David, Star and Crescent, Om, or Ahimsa hand).

Critical Thinking Questions: What additional discoveries have I made during this activity? What additional information would be helpful for me to include?

The health of a community is heavily influenced by local religious institutions in the organization of services and as vehicles of social and economic support for their members. Although many of the earlier direct-care functions have disappeared, some religious groups remain strong community advocates for health and bring considerable cultural capital to the public health table for migrant health, senior citizen–health promotion, care of preschool children, neighborhood improvement, and school-violence abatement. The Catholic Church, for example, is the largest provider of nongovernment healthcare and education in the United States. Faith-based philanthropies, such as Jewish Federation and Catholic Charities, provide substantial community benefit to underserved populations and are important private-sector partners with local public health departments.

Many religious institutions play a significant role in reducing health disparities with funds, equipment, and health and social-support services, such as cooking and housekeeping, disease prevention, and health-promotion activities. Even if they do not participate directly, religious institutions often lend their facilities to community health services, such as after-school programs for teenagers, child day care centers, senior centers, and sites for health fairs. Like other institutions, organized religions not only have buildings and activities; they have leaders and officials who are likely to have considerable influence in the community and can support particular health projects. Religions are key institutions for resolving community health problems (Peterson, Atwood, & Yates, 2002).

Prevailing religious beliefs involving diet, pregnancy, family planning, and terminal illness must be considered in the development of community health education and programming. Furthermore, certain religions may impose injunctions on common public health screening or prevention procedures. Finally, the relationship between religiosity and mortality, suggested more than 30 years ago in the Alameda County Study by Lisa Berkman and Leonard Syme (1979), has been confirmed, with continued lower mortality rates for frequent attendees of religious services. This correlation appears to be explained by improved health practices, increased social contact, and more stable marriages (Strawbridge, Cohen, Shema, & Kaplan, 1997) as well as more emotional support, a sense of spiritual connectedness, optimism, and better health in old age (Krause, 2002).

Education

Suggested Activity

Do the following:

- Describe the local governance of the public school system.
- Identify pre-college-level schools—including public, alternative, and private—that serve the population, and locate them on the map.
- Determine the number of families who homeschool their children.
- Determine the approximate enrollment in each school or program.
- Describe the administration of the local public school system, including the following:
    - The function of the school board
    - The composition of the school board
    - How board members are elected or appointed
- Describe how the superintendent of schools is selected.
- List the names of the principal of each school.
- Describe the function and role of the school nurse. For example, how many people (children and school personnel) is the school nurse responsible for? Who are the ancillary personnel assisting with the care of the children? What type of training do school personnel receive to manage medication and health concerns when the nurse is not available?
- Describe other health services, including health and physical education curricula, offered through the schools.
- What kinds of special services are available for children with physical and mental disabilities?
- Identify the educational institutions that are used for adult learning in the community.

> ▪ Identify the libraries and other educational facilities available to community residents.
>
> Critical Thinking Questions: What additional discoveries have I made during this activity? What additional information would be helpful for me to include?

The local school is a vital influence in the life of the child and family, and the school system is an essential component of a community's cultural capital. In addition to traditional screening in the form of physical, vision, and hearing exams, the school system provides free and reduced lunches and some breakfasts for low-income children as well as after-school care. School nurses work with trained ancillary personnel to manage acute and chronic health conditions and engage in health promotion, with educational and screening programs for such issues as depression, drug abuse, sex education, dental health, vision, nutrition, and hygiene. Some schools also provide primary care with school-based health clinics staffed by nurse practitioners, offering healthcare for low-income and uninsured children who may otherwise encounter barriers to healthcare services.

Many schools have a strong sense of community and are the setting for family fun nights and health fairs where children as well as their families can learn about health-related topics together. Schools maintain information about the numbers of children receiving free and reduced lunches, which helps identify pockets of low-income families who may have greater needs for health surveillance and services. School records on absenteeism provide an excellent source of data for case-finding and epidemiological investigations. Developing relationships with the principal, school secretary, and teachers of each school creates a foundation for efficiently reaching the majority of children and families in a community. Many states mandate the employment of a school nurse at the elementary and secondary levels. The role of the school nurse encompasses the totality of the school-health program, incorporating primary, secondary, and tertiary prevention strategies and creating a healthy school environment that provides a safe, supportive social environment and learning milieu for all children.

School boards differ in the degree of influence they exert on schools. Some retain great control over every aspect of school life, while others leave the administration to the principal and limit their input to financial matters. The composition and philosophy of the board influence school health programs. In addition to getting to know the principal and teachers, it is valuable to meet the board members, especially those with a known interest in health topics, to enlist their support in building community capacity.

Adult-education classes have become increasingly popular and provide an effective mechanism for offering health-related courses, such as CPR and emergency care, parenting, and stress reduction. Expert faculty members can assume a leadership role in promoting a healthy community agenda. The effectiveness of our schools and colleges and the ability of public health workers to reach all members of the community are central to public health.

Recreation

Play and recreation are important components of all societies. Recreation is directly related to health in its capacity for providing exercise, for meeting physical and psychological challenges, and for offering relaxation and stress relief. The promotion of organized recreational activities, such as at supervised playgrounds and parks, has been a significant public health intervention for reducing accidents and promoting the safety of children. Recreation generates social interaction in the form of teams and clubs that can break down barriers and create the sense of unity that symbolizes a healthy community.

Recreation also can also be engaged in by taking time to relax and enjoy books, magazines, radio, television, and the Internet. These recreational activities also serve a communication function and are important resources for public health education, particularly in the area of health promotion, prevention of disease, and personal management of health problems. The Internet provides ready access to a range of health information and rapid communication. Practically all women's and family magazines have health columns. Television shows, movies, soap operas, and novels deal with a variety of health problems, including driving while intoxicated, teenage suicide, drug abuse, family violence, living with chronic illness, Alzheimer's disease, and death and dying. Sensitively written and framed within the cultural experience of the audience, they can be valuable teaching tools as well as vehicles for mobilizing community action (for example, through a community reading program). The timing of health education or health-screening programs to immediately follow a television drama that has generated the interest of the public can help ensure its success.

Suggested Activity
Do the following:

- Describe how community residents spend their leisure time.
- Locate and identify recreational areas and facilities. These include formal recreation facilities (e.g., parks, playgrounds, theaters, zoos, golf courses, public pools) and informal recreational facilities (e.g., streets, vacant lots, swimming holes).
- Describe the quality, accessibility, and use of recreational facilities.
- Locate publicly supported facilities, commercial facilities, and/or age-designated facilities (e.g., for children, adolescents, senior citizens).
- Describe where children go to play.
- Note the times of the day and the week generally reserved for leisure activity.
- List the agencies and personnel specifically concerned with community recreation and leisure.

Critical Thinking Questions: What additional discoveries have I made during this activity? What additional information would be helpful for me to include?

Although recreational and leisure facilities offer distinct advantages for the purpose of promoting the health and safety of community residents, they can also generate community health problems. Excessive alcohol consumption or a "binge-drinking culture," for example, can have serious consequences for communities.

The safety and sanitation of public recreational facilities is another component of community practice. Broken bottles and rusty cans left in the park or on a beach can cause serious injuries. Some leisure and play activities place the participants at risk of personal injury and therefore require appropriate community resources to prevent and manage potential injuries. Although individuals and groups should not be prevented from the pleasures of mountain climbing, motorcycle riding, driving ATVs, scuba diving, running marathons, cycling, and playing football, they all carry considerable risk for injury and cost that may be borne by the community. Such sports as boating, snowmobiling, skiing, or skating may require public health–initiated regulations, injury-prevention programs, and trauma services.

Voluntary Associations

Suggested Activity

Do the following:

- Identify the voluntary organizations in the community by type:
  - Social
  - Economic
  - Religious
  - Educational
  - Political
  - Recreational
- Identify the leaders of each organization.
- Identify when, where, and how often they meet.
- Identify informal associations and groups within the community.

Critical Thinking Questions: What additional discoveries have I made during this activity? What additional information would be helpful for me to include?

A culturally acceptable and efficient way to establish partnerships for action is to engage existing community groups. Voluntary associations are very important assets in a community to help in building community capacity. They represent strength in leadership and membership that can be readily deployed by community/public health nurses to solve community problems and promote community health. Each of the institutions already discussed has its own voluntary associations consisting of groups of individuals who are bound together by a common interest. Therefore, there are many kinds of voluntary associations based on their stated purposes. One category, for example, consists of those based on common socio-demographic characteristics, such as age (teen groups, young adults), ethnicity (Polish American clubs, Sons of Cuba), and attendance at the same school (alumni associations, fraternities and sororities). Often, local branch associations are tied into national organizations and are highly formalized, such as the Masons or Elks clubs. Organizations that are national or international in scope are important resources for obtaining support from outside the community.

Typical economic voluntary associations are the chamber of commerce, trade associations, professional societies, or Kiwanis clubs. Occupational groups form to control and oversee various aspects of their trades or professions. Government and political associations, political-party branch organizations, and citizens' councils, such as the League of Women Voters, usually function to influence legislation locally and/or nationally. Voluntary associations also provide protective services, such as fire and police protection. Parent-teacher associations are perhaps the best-known of all educational voluntary associations, but others include voluntary library services and bookmobiles as well as travel societies, book clubs, and honor societies. Organized religion has led the way in establishing voluntary associations to carry on community activities. Church brotherhoods or women's committees, the YMCA, the YWCA, B'nai B'rith, and Jewish community centers are all examples of religious voluntary associations. Many recreational and artistic activities also are organized on a voluntary basis, including athletic clubs, choruses, bridge clubs, dance and theater groups, and chamber-music ensembles.

Voluntary groups ordinarily are formalized with titles and charters, regular meetings, and criteria for membership. Other groups are more informally organized but equally important. These include teenagers who routinely meet in the local shopping mall, elders who eat breakfast at the same restaurant every morning, and men who gather each evening on a street corner or play chess in the park. Even though such informal groups are more difficult to identify and appear to be leaderless, they may have even more community influence than formal groups and provide a constituency that could lend valuable support in creating and implementing a culturally informed healthy community agenda.

Practically all voluntary associations serve functions beyond their stated purposes, including lobbying politicians or helping members acquire jobs or borrow money. In addition, holding offices in voluntary organizations gives people a chance to pursue leadership opportunities and attain status. Many join voluntary associations as a form of recreation, even if the goals of the association are not recreational. Voluntary associations also help newcomers to the community fit in and meet others with similar interests. Voluntary associations provide social guidance, imposing injunctions on the behavior of members and requiring that they conform to specific standards. Alcoholics Anonymous, for example, and other self-help groups have blossomed into a panorama of mutual assistance and support, gaining public attention for addressing such health problems as obesity, smoking, cancer, muscular dystrophy, diabetes, and Alzheimer's disease. Many groups focused on health issues and problems were inspired and organized on the local level by nurses who recognized that affected individuals could relate to and learn from others with the same problems, knowing they had undergone similar experiences.

HORIZONTAL DIVISIONS OF THE COMMUNITY

Differences in wealth and status exist in practically all communities, no matter how small and homogeneous they first appear. These differences, when examined at the population level, constitute social classes of people that correlate more or less closely with income, educational level, and occupation. *Social class* represents categories of people of similar social rank having positions, responsibilities, possessions, and accomplishments of a more or less equal level and value.

Suggested Activity

Do the following:

- Describe the major socioeconomic levels in the community.
- Identify the socio-demographic variables and social institutions that distinguish these levels.

Critical Thinking Questions: What additional discoveries have I made during this activity? What additional information would be helpful for me to include?

For those who are unfamiliar with a particular community, patterns of class stratification and socioeconomic differences between residents may be barely distinguishable, particularly if all citizens in the community have limited access to resources. Residents will often deny the existence of social classes in their communities. Even so, the recognition of socioeconomic differences is of critical importance in understanding the community's social structure and power relationships. The differences that exist on the community level may not always—in fact, often do not—reflect the class differences that exist on the national level. They are nevertheless consequential for the community and are acknowledged by community members.

Most residents have an awareness of their position in relation to others. It is difficult to find a community where differences in status, income, and access to scarce resources do not exist. Even though social classes are not formally organized groups, like voluntary associations, they have lives of their own. People enter them through birth or marriage or, with some difficulty, through the acquisition of socioeconomic resources and power as they progress through life. Although there is no formal membership process for entering a class, to be counted among a specific rank requires that others judge you to be so. This acceptance often is more difficult to obtain than the more formal membership of voluntary associations.

Generally, it is assumed that income, family name, occupation, residence, and education guide the social ranking of individuals. This is not always the case, however, as the criteria for determining social rank vary from community to community. Any member of the community may assume symbols of high social status, such as manner of dress, etiquette, residence, and car, but these symbols do not mean the person is actually a member of that class. Moreover, the upper echelons as well as members of this individual's own social rank may criticize him or her for trying to imitate those of a higher social rank. Nor can one assume that wealth and a profession will automatically qualify a resident for a particular social class. Although the actual ranking of individuals or households in terms of their socioeconomic status is not within the scope of this book, we can learn much about the culture of a community simply by the way people group themselves for social interaction—particularly in the areas of recreation and education. Because friendships and social activities often tend to follow class lines, the task of delineating socioeconomic strata for a particular community is not as difficult as one may anticipate. Church memberships may embrace a wide range of social levels, and the workplace may include all ranks present in the community, but it is less likely that people of different classes will socialize routinely. The presence of private schools in a community along with the public school system also provide some clues as to how individuals rank themselves and each other. The horizontal division of the community reveals the most fundamental power structure of the community. The support of people in the upper strata of the community is extremely helpful in accessing certain kinds of cultural-capital and building-community capacity. The same people, however, also can pose serious obstacles or threats to community health action.

VERTICAL DIVISIONS OF THE COMMUNITY

In contrast to horizontal divisions of a community, vertical divisions are those sectors in the community that are not necessarily related to socioeconomic status or classes but that nevertheless organize the community into subgroups. Depending on the community, these could be organized according to racial, ethnic, residential, religious, political, or occupational factors. A familiar example of vertical division of a community is the urban neighborhood composed of two or more dominant subgroups—such as Irish and Italian or African American and Puerto Rican—each of which may or may not express a full range of class or socioeconomic differentiation. Even though they may live side by side, the two groups may vote for different political candidates, have different social clubs, participate in different recreational activities, belong to different religions, and enjoy different family lifestyles. Although they may intermingle on a daily basis, when there is a dispute between representatives of the two factions, it is likely they will support their respective groups.

Suggested Activity

Do the following:

- Identify the vertical divisions of the community by type.
- Describe them in terms of differences in their institutions and socio-demographic characteristics.

Critical Thinking Questions: What additional discoveries have I made during this activity? What additional information would be helpful for me to include?

Although people within these diverse segments share a common affiliation, they are rarely homogeneous, with social class, age, and religious differences prompting differences in values and lifestyles. Segment boundaries are permeated through marriage and childbearing so that some residents eventually claim membership in more than one social segment. These are important residents, because they often have influence that spans the whole community. Such vertical divisions are not limited to ethnic groups. Communities may be divided by such characteristics as residence (apartment dwellers, homeowners, and homeless), politics (Republicans, Democrats, and Independents), or religion (Christians, Jews, and Muslims). Traditional conflicts between farmers and ranchers suggest similar factions based on occupation and the competition for land and water. In some cases, vertical divisions in a community are not easily discovered and only become evident in times of conflict.

Similar to classes, vertical divisions in a community may not be formally organized groups in the sense of having regular charters, membership status, formal leadership, explicit rules of behavior, or routine meetings. Rather, they arise when a group of citizens has something in common that differentiates them from another group within the community. Despite the lack of officers, a charismatic leader is often heartily endorsed by other members of the group, someone who is highly persuasive, has the ability to sway large numbers of people, and influences citizen action, including elections.

For many people, the term *community* implies relationships of equality among its members. This discussion of social organization clearly shows that communities are, in fact, complex entities, made up not just of an environment and people but also of diverse institutions, classes, and groups with interests and goals that are sometimes shared and sometimes in conflict. It is important to know which segments of the community can be counted on to support a particular project and which cannot. It also is important to know which themes and activities unite community residents of various classes and segments and which separate them. It may be difficult, for example, to change public policy unless all the dominant segments of a multicultural community support the effort. The strategies for mobilizing citizen action for capacity building are discussed in Chapter 7, "Laying the Foundation for a Healthy Community Agenda," and Chapter 8, "Leading Culturally Informed Community Action."

Unlike the tangible physical environment and unlike people, we cannot always see or touch a class, an institution, or a vertical division of a community. A series of diagrams depicting the horizontal and vertical divisions of a community in relation to each other and to community institutions can be very helpful to illustrate the social system and its points of intersection and cleavage. If, for example, the class structure were diagrammed according to religious institutions, it might be found that in some communities, all social levels attend the same church. This would thus be a *point of intersection* in the community—that is, a place where the nurse could reach a broad range of community residents as opposed to a specific segment.

Suggested Activity

Diagram the horizontal and vertical divisions of your community to look for points of intersection and points of separation, as in the following example.

Horizontal Divisions in a Small Town with a Single-Purpose Economy

Stratum	Religion	Economy	Schools	Recreation	Domestic	Housing
Upper elite	Catholic Anglican	Factory owner Professional Business	Private schools Catholic schools	Tennis Golf Sports fans Health clubs	Nuclear Older couples Single parent	Owners Large single family
Middle class	Methodist Catholic Baptist	Managers Commercial Teachers Government Trades	Public schools Catholic schools Private schools	Camping Sports fans Running	Nuclear Single parent	Owners Renters New tract housing
Working class	Catholic	Factory workers Unemployed	Public schools Catholic schools	Bowling league Sports fans	Large extended Single parent	Owners Renters

Vertical Divisions in an Urban Community Undergoing Gentrification

Institution	Indigenous Sicilian Families	Newcomers
Religion	Catholic	Various religions
Economy	Dock workers	Business people working out of neighborhood
	Local merchants	
	Hospital workers	Artists
	Trades	
Education	High school	Professional degrees
	Trade schools	College graduates
Recreation	Eastside bars	Westside clubs
Family	Large, extended, relatives nearby	Single person
		Couples and one-child families
Housing (city brownstones)	Owners	Renters/owners

Even though the community's health status has not been addressed directly, simply looking at its environment, its people, and the ways in which people are organized and relate to their environment can help you identify many potential problems and concerns. This inquiry into the culture of a community not only exposes current health problems and predicts future ones; it also reveals the assets, strengths, and cultural capital that can be activated through citizen participation to build community capacity in the most culturally informed way.

DETERMINING THE HEALTH OF YOUR COMMUNITY

A healthy community is grounded in a wholesome environment, promotes social justice and inclusiveness, and prevents and responds to health risks and problems in a timely and culturally informed manner. This chapter provides a systematic format for assessing the health of a community's environment, the population, and the effectiveness of the ideological and institutional health organizations available to address health concerns and create a healthy community.

CHAPTER 6 OBJECTIVES

- Learn to describe and analyze the health of a community.

- Apply a systematic process and comprehensive framework to assess the health of a community.

- Compare the health of a community in different time periods and with other communities.

- Examine a community's healthcare resources and accessibility to them in terms of primary, secondary, and tertiary prevention.

- Examine the range of local beliefs and values related to health and healing.

COMMUNITY HEALTH ASSESSMENT

The community health assessment complements and completes the community culture inquiry, documenting not only the community's needs but also the resources available to accomplish the goals of *Healthy People 2020*. Communities are dynamic organizations in which the strengths and the opportunities for improvement are constantly changing. Like the examination of community culture, the community health assessment is an ongoing process of documenting, comparing, and analyzing environmental, population, and health-organization indicators. Similar to the community culture inquiry framework discussed in Chapter 5, "Discovering the Culture of Your Community," the community health assessment in this chapter is organized according to environment, population, and social organization—specifically, the organization of health and healthcare. The community health assessment framework provided in this chapter is not exhaustive. Depending on the community, some components of the assessment will be more or less useful than others. Also, in some cases, additional kinds of information may be needed to better understand and address community health issues, problems, and the resources available to address them. We encourage you to use the resources listed in Chapter 4 as well as the *Healthy People 2020* website to supplement your review of community health statistics and resources as you complete your community health assessment. As you complete the assessment, consider whether and how the community is able to meet the health needs of target populations who are disproportionately affected by their vulnerabilities, such as the effects of poverty, low literacy, migrant status, or age (e.g., very young, adolescents, and elders). Remember, it is important to meet with members of the community to gain their perspectives. Key informants, community stakeholders, healthcare professionals, focus groups, and trusted laypersons knowledgeable about the community all have valuable insights to offer.

ENVIRONMENTAL HEALTH

The culture inquiry in Chapter 5 identified topographical, meteorological, and climatic features of the environment that may offer protection from, or place a community at risk for, widespread health problems. Urbanization; the invention of the automobile, telephone, and computers; and the development of nuclear technology have drastically altered the temporal and spatial dimensions of cultures throughout the world. Rapid changes over the past two centuries have intensified global warming and pollution and necessitated greater public health action.

Ensuring the health of a community requires ensuring the health of the environment. In the aftermath of a natural disaster, such as the earthquake and the subsequent cholera outbreak in Haiti in 2010, departures from environmental standards for cleanliness and safety precipitated serious health problems and compromised the most essential requirements to sustain life—air, water, and food—as the disaster affected dwellings, the workplace, communication, and transportation. Improving the quality of the environment improves the health of residents and the relationships among them. *Healthy People 2020* includes environmental health as one of its major topic areas with the following six themes:

- Outdoor air quality

- Surface and groundwater quality

- Toxic substances and hazardous waste

- Homes and communities

- Infrastructure and surveillance

- Global environmental health

The influence of the environment is not a new topic in public health (Armelagos, Brown, & Turner, 2005). Natural forces, such as volcanoes, dust storms, weather depressions, floods, and insect pests, have altered air, water, and food supplies in ways that have threatened human life. Over the centuries, humans have burned wood and charcoal, causing localized air pollution. In 2014, the urban global population was estimated at 54% and expected to grow approximately 1.84% per year between 2015 and 2020 (World Health Organization [WHO], 2015). This process of urbanization has most likely placed the environment at greatest risk. Pollution and cities go hand in hand as dense populations of people strain the environment. Overcrowding and environmental overload exhaust environmental resources, and high-density populations often are associated with industrial activity that adulterates soil, water, and air with various forms of solid and gaseous contaminants. Foul odors, dirty streets and roads, unkempt housing, and unclean recreational areas all give the impression of a population that has lost interest in the place where its members live, work, and play. The effects can be dismal and may promote a negativism that pervades the community. On the other hand, a beautiful environment that is uncluttered and pleasing to the senses is not only a signal but also a source of community health.

Safeguarding the environment for the health of the public is an international challenge. Even remote contamination sites affect communities located thousands of miles away. In 2011, when the nuclear facilities in Japan were damaged as a result of an earthquake and the ensuing tsunami, all the local residents were removed from the area around the power plants, and citizens on the West Coast of the United States also took precautions against contamination. This is an example of how the detrimental effects of the tsunami on environmental health in a small community in northern Japan may generate health risks in national and global arenas. There have been repeated attempts at international collaboration to promote sustainable means to lower the levels of carbon-dioxide emissions, manage the production and storage of nuclear waste, limit worldwide population growth to sustainable levels, and address the economic inequities that plague the world environment. These four factors are implicated in the self-perpetuating cycle of ecological degradation found worldwide (Friedman, 2008).

The environmental assessment parameters provided here are intended as a framework and are by no means exhaustive. Rather, they can be used as a guide to some of the most common environmental health problems. The relevance and prioritization of problems will vary from community to community. Industrialized societies, for example, will be concerned with nuclear contamination, while agricultural communities may be more concerned with soil contamination, pesticide runoff, insect control, and potable water.

OUTDOOR AIR QUALITY

Suggested Activity

Do the following:

- Record the air-quality index of the community.
- Describe the measures being put into place to reduce the risk of adverse health effects caused by air pollution.
- Identify the actual and potential sources of air pollution.
- List the major modes of transportation in the community.
- Identify the topographical or climatic features that contribute to air pollution.
- Describe indications of outdoor air quality (e.g., smells, dense air pollution, or people wearing face masks).
- List local health problems that are attributable to air pollution.
- Show the trends over the past 20 years regarding air pollution.
- Compare these trends to state, national, and international levels.
- Identify the populations disproportionately affected by air pollution.

Critical Thinking Questions: What additional discoveries have I made during this activity? What additional information would be helpful to include?

The quality of the outdoor air is a major factor in promoting the health and survival of the human community. Exposure to air pollution contributes to a variety of health problems, such as asthma, emphysema, lung cancer, bronchitis, pneumonia, cardiopulmonary disease, chronic obstructive pulmonary disease (COPD), and other chronic lung diseases. Although most health problems associated with air pollution affect the respiratory system, eye irritation and dermatological reactions also are common.

Air pollution is a result of contamination of the atmosphere by airborne substances that are potentially harmful to humans as well as to animals and plants. For centuries, people have burned wood and its derivatives for cooking and for heat, thus emitting ash, smoke, soot, and dust into the air. It was during the Industrial Revolution in England, however, that contamination of the air received the greatest attention from public health officials, inspiring movements to regulate the burning of coal to control the amount of smoke and soot. Polluting particulate matter has expanded from the derivatives of wood to include aerosol droplets, pesticides, insecticides, and herbicides. Cigarette smoking, traditionally considered a personal-health problem, has now assumed significance as a public health problem, as research has confirmed that the noxious components of tobacco smoke are damaging not only to those who smoke but also to those who are exposed to secondhand smoke. Approximately 58% of the population in the United States lives in communities where outdoor air-pollution levels are dangerous to health, with persons in poverty at higher risk (American Lung Association, 2010). The respiratory consequences of air pollution are mediated by the weather. Acid aerosols are worse in the winter in areas where coal-fired industry is common. Oxidates, including atmospheric ozone, are worse in the summer, especially from midday to late afternoon, when the sun is the hottest.

Today, the major sources of air pollution are emissions from motor vehicles, agricultural production (animal and plant), industry, and energy production. The emission of noxious gases, such as carbon monoxide, carbon dioxide, and sulfur dioxide from petroleum and coal combustion, and chlorofluorocarbons (CFCs) from propellant spray cans, solvents, and refrigerants, has also contributed to contamination of the air. These gases are hypothesized to contribute to an intensified greenhouse effect by depleting ozone in the stratosphere, which provides a vital protective layer against lethal irradiation. If the predicted global warming resulting from the increase in greenhouse gases actually takes place, the consequences for health and human survival could be catastrophic (Centers for Disease Control and Prevention, 2015).

Although controversy about the timing, cause, and extent of climate change continues, there is little debate about its effect on rainfall, groundwater, food production, and ozone depletion. Topographical factors and climatic conditions interact with sources of air pollution to create even more pernicious and widespread problems. Mexico City, Denver, and Los Angeles, for example, have particularly serious problems because of topographical features that trap polluted air over the most populated areas. Communities that lie in a river valley often are subject to *air inversion*—that is, the trapping of warm air on the ground by cooler air higher up, a common occurrence in valley ecologies. It is not unusual for the level of air pollution in such communities to be incompatible with national standards.

SURFACE- AND GROUNDWATER QUALITY

Suggested Activity

Do the following:

- Identify the proportion of people in the community who consume water that meets the standards set in the Safe Drinking Water Act.
- Identify the source of the public water supply.
- Find out the proportion of households using private water supplies.
- Describe the process that is used to treat the water supply.
- Report the frequency of water supply inspections.
- Identify unsatisfactory water reports over the past 5 years.
- Locate on a map and date episodes of outbreaks of disease due to water pollution over the past 5 years.
- Report industrial or human waste being discharged into local water.
- Describe fluoridation policies.
- Identify the populations disproportionately affected by water pollution.

Critical Thinking Questions: What additional discoveries have I made during this activity? What additional information would be helpful to include?

A safe and adequate water supply is essential to the health and survival of a population. With development, redistribution of waterways, and contamination of groundwater, water has been called "global gold" and is an underlying cause of wars and social injustices. From early times, water has been essential to life and also a means to dispose of waste. Communities may pollute rivers, streams, and lakes with sewage disposal and industrial byproducts, contaminating the water sources of communities downstream. In most industrialized societies, the bacteriologic infections carried by water, such as cholera, have been greatly reduced or eliminated through water-treatment processes, including the addition of chlorides. The potential for pollution of surface and groundwater by industrial waste, however—including radioactive materials and lethal chemical byproducts—is cause for concern.

An environmental assessment to ensure the drinkability—or potability—of water includes the public water supply and private springs or wells. Affecting every continent, water scarcity and inadequate sanitation are an increasing global concern (United Nations Department of Economic and Social Affairs, 2010). Scarcity of water resources affects 2.8 billion people for at least 1 month in a calendar year, with more than 1.2 billion persons lacking access to clean water on a regular basis. The causes are multifactorial and include climate change, overuse of freshwater resources, and depletion of natural resources (United Nations Department of Economic and Social Affairs, 2010). Additionally, lack of sanitation causes such diseases as cholera, dysentery, and other diarrheal problems, a leading cause of childhood mortality. Clean water supplies also are important for recreation, such as swimming and boating, and commerce, such as fishing. The addition of chemicals to the public water supply has been a much-debated public health issue, particularly with reference to fluorides. On the other hand, the increase in dental-health problems due to unfluoridated water supplies is also a public health problem. A *Healthy People 2020* recommendation is to increase the percentage of the population served by community water systems, identifying households not using the public water supply as at higher risk for dental-health problems. Herbicides and pesticides used in agriculture also are potentially harmful pollutants, and water in such communities, as well as those bordering and downstream, require testing specifically for these products.

FOOD CONTAMINATION

Suggested Activity

Do the following:

- Locate and date outbreaks or episodes of illness as a result of unsanitary or adulterated food products. What causative organisms are identified (e.g., salmonella, listeria)? How many people were affected by the outbreaks?

- Identify causative factors leading to outbreaks of disease, such as undercooked foods, poor refrigeration, globalization and transportation of food products, or contamination from animal or human feces.

- Identify pesticides and herbicides used to protect local food crops.

- Identify the use of antibiotics in the production of food products from animal sources and the effects they have on human health.

- Identify food-garden sites located near contaminated water, soil, or air.

- Identify populations disproportionately affected by food contamination.

- Which public health measures exist to prevent food contamination and protect food sources (e.g., restaurant inspections)?

Critical Thinking Questions: What additional discoveries have I made during this activity? What additional information would be helpful to include?

Food contamination can be caused by a variety of pollutants in the air, water, or soil. Dumping dangerous chemical waste products pollutes water and contaminates local fish products. The use of pesticides and herbicides is a threat to those who handle them, and downstream water supplies are often toxic. DDT, which used to be one of the most commonly used pesticides, is so toxic that it was banned in the early 1970s. Public health concerns over outbreaks of infection from food and milk contamination have now shifted to problems created by the adulteration of artificial food products. In addition to chemical fertilizers, the purposeful addition of other nonfood ingredients to enhance the flavor, augment the color, increase the size, and improve the shelf life of a product all are examples of food adulteration, whose impact on health is only partially known.

TOXIC SUBSTANCES AND HAZARDOUS WASTE MANAGEMENT

The ability to create a safe and healthful environment for a flourishing community requires the management of various forms of contaminants and other hazardous wastes, such as sewage, solid waste, lead, chemical and pesticide byproducts, and radioactive materials. Uncontrolled dumping of waste poses a serious threat to the air, water, and food necessary to support human life and the aesthetics to enhance it.

Solid Waste

The unintentional consequences of modern living have resulted in disposable and nonbiodegradable materials, which can be found in the litter of bottles, plastic grocery bags, cans, and plastic containers that pollute the land and seascapes. The collection and disposal of solid wastes and unwanted byproducts of industry are major public health problems, not only because of the potential contamination of water and food supplies but also because of the risk to animals and the unsightliness of the environment. Foul-smelling and rat-infested dumps create a health and an aesthetic problem for community residents. As landfills reach capacity, financial and political controversies have emerged. It is not unusual for residents to oppose new plans for solid waste–disposal sites. Illegal dumping has become a criminal activity but often falls outside the control of local public health authorities.

Suggested Activity

Do the following:

- Identify sources of solid wastes.
- Describe where and how solid wastes are disposed and/or recycled.
- Record community health problems within the past 5 years as a result of solid wastes.
- Describe compliance of solid waste–disposal with federal, state, and local regulations.
- Map and date public recreational facilities (parks, campgrounds, or beaches) condemned within the last 5 years as a result of solid-waste dumping.
- Map breaches of sanitary codes in the last 5 years.
- Map areas where disposal of trash and garbage is a visible problem.

Critical Thinking Questions: What additional discoveries have I made during this activity? What additional information would be helpful to include?

Sewage

Every culture and community has firmly established patterns for the disposal of human wastes and the management of fecal materials. As with other forms of pollution, urbanization has limited the facilities available for adequate sewage disposal in densely populated settlements. Rural communities also require vigilance regarding the management of human waste. Septic tanks and cesspools are used in rural areas for waste disposal and inspected regularly. As with other forms of waste, the management of sewage has health and aesthetic implications. Waterborne diseases, such as *Giardia*, cholera, and amebiasis, are the direct result of contamination by animal or human fecal material.

Suggested Activity

Do the following:

- Describe local methods for eliminating sewage.

- Identify local cultural practices and beliefs related to the elimination of fecal waste.

- Identify sources of sewage contamination in the environment.

- Describe sewage-management compliance with local, state, and federal codes.

- Map and date outbreaks of disease or other health problems attributed to problems with sewage management during the last 5 years.

- Identify populations disproportionately affected by sewage contamination.

Critical Thinking Questions: What additional discoveries have I made during this activity? What additional information would be helpful to include?

Radioactive Waste

Although millions of contaminants, in certain quantities, can be damaging to the health of a population, radioactive substances probably have received the most attention in recent years, particularly as the need for energy increases. Everyone is exposed to some form of radiation simply through natural contact with the cosmic rays of the sun and substances of Earth. Radon is being recognized as a naturally occurring source that increases risk for lung cancer. More dangerous levels of exposure come from medical X-rays, uranium mining and processing, nuclear power plants, and nuclear-weapons development. The production, transportation, storage, and disposal of radioactive materials, such as nuclear fuel, present a significant health and safety hazard. Furthermore, the contamination of groundwater supplies can spread the danger far beyond the local community. Since the development of the nuclear-weapons industry at the end of World War II, radioactive materials have been released into our environment.

Suggested Activity

Do the following:

- Identify on a map the location of regional nuclear power plants.

- Map documented radioactive contamination in the community. What is the source of the contamination (e.g., naturally occurring, such as radon, as well as man-made)?

- Describe the community's role in the transport, storage, and/or disposal of radioactive materials.

- Describe the level of compliance in the management of radioactive materials with federal and state regulations.

- Map public health problems attributable to nuclear/radioactive exposure within the last 5 years.

- Compare rates of cancer, particularly leukemia, to state and national rates.

- Describe social or psychological problems associated with nuclear exposure.

- Identify populations disproportionately exposed to radiation.

- Identify measures to assess indoor air quality for those who live in high-risk areas.

Critical Thinking Questions: What additional discoveries have I made during this activity? What additional information would be helpful to include?

The disposal of nuclear waste, given the long half-life of many of its toxic products, is a foremost public health concern and, in the event of a nuclear meltdown, a crisis. Various states have raised objections in Congress to the mass transfer of nuclear waste to be stored within their borders. As with other forms of waste, cases of illegal dumping of nuclear material place the public at risk in spite of government regulation. The potential for sabotage and accidents in the storage and transport of nuclear materials poses physical and psychological threats. Many health risks are associated with exposure to radiation, including leukemia and other forms of cancer, genetic mutations, and fetal damage. Careful records reporting the incidence of such diseases and health problems from year to year provide important data regarding potential radioactive contamination.

Chemicals and Pesticides

Suggested Activity

Do the following:

- Map sources of chemicals and pesticides in the community.
- Identify the percentage of children with elevated blood-lead levels.
- Determine how many healthcare provider visits are attributable to chemical and pesticide exposure.
- Describe the compliance of chemical and pesticide management with federal and state guidelines.
- Identify evidence of uncontrolled or illegal dumping.
- Identify health problems or outbreaks of disease attributed to chemicals and pesticides in the last 5 years.
- Identify social or psychological problems attributed to exposure to chemicals and pesticides.
- Map nearby Superfund sites.
- Identify populations that are disproportionately exposed to chemicals and pesticides.
- Interview local residents regarding their personal use and disposal of chemicals and pesticides in the home environment.
- Map community locations for residents to safely dispose of toxic chemicals and pesticides.

Critical Thinking Questions: What additional discoveries have I made during this activity? What additional information would be helpful to include?

Although it was not a new problem, the pollution of the environment from dangerous chemical waste first received serious public attention with the Love Canal incident in the early 1970s (Levine, 1982). Hazardous chemicals were leaching from an abandoned disposal site located in an old canal where an elementary school had been built. Because the disposal had begun in the 1940s and was decades old, most residents of this newly thriving community in upstate New York were unaware of the disposal site's proximity to the area where their homes were built. After families had moved into their homes, the chemical pollution traveled through underground waterways into yards and basements and vaporized into the air. After extensive media attention and political involvement, studies were conducted that revealed an excessive miscarriage rate among the population, although other health risks were not so definitively implicated. Many people moved their families from this site, and many more became aware of the difficulty of addressing suspected environmental problems (Newton & Smith, 2004).

Similar problems were encountered with Agent Orange, a defoliant used during the Vietnam War. Exposure to chemical-warfare agents in Iraq during Operation Desert Storm was suspected of causing health problems, which the press dubbed "Gulf War Syndrome." The uncontrolled dumping of chemical wastes through the 20th century and the illegal dumping of more recent years continue to pose major health problems for the nation. The National Priorities List, also known as the *Superfund sites,* scores hazardous-waste sites by a hazard-ranking system. More than 1,400 Superfund sites are located in the United States, and the Agency for Toxic Substances and Disease Registry (ATSDR) assesses their potential for health effects. Congress established this federal program, designed to clean up huge sites of chemical, nuclear, and industrial waste, in 1980. The Environmental Protection Agency (EPA) designates Superfund sites.

Each day, new research findings implicate exposure to dangerous chemicals and pesticides as the etiology of many health problems, including various forms of cancer, birth defects, neurological disorders, reproductive problems, immunological disturbances, gastrointestinal problems, dermatological diseases, and vision problems (*Healthy People 2020*). For example, human exposure to lead can cause such problems as hypertension, anemia, kidney damage, learning disabilities, and impaired fetal development. Increased levels of lead in the environment occur from the corrosion of leaded water pipes as well as from man-made products, such as car batteries, cables, pipelines, lead-based paints, tainted candy wrappers, pesticides, ceramic glazes, candles, cigarette smoke, and the glass in computer and television screens. Although we know about the hazardous effects of lead, only roughly 20% of the approximately 60,000 industrial chemicals used in this country have been tested for their toxic potential to human health. Sources of exposure include water contamination, lawn fertilizers, contaminated food and dairy products, pesticides and herbicides, and some disinfectants. In a study of 270 pregnant women, detectable levels of 163 chemicals were found in 100% of the women, and perchlorate (a regulated chemical used in propellants for rockets and explosives) was found in 99% to 100% of the women (Woodruff, Zota, & Schwartz, 2011). The exposure of pregnant and lactating women, infants, and young children to these products is thought to be correlated with birth defects and blood disorders, including leukemia. *Healthy People 2020* recommends monitoring blood and urine to measure the recommended reduced exposure to such chemicals as arsenic, cadmium, lead, mercury, chlordane, DDT, and others. It is critically important not only to monitor the effects of hazardous chemicals but also to advocate for their removal.

NOISE POLLUTION

An often-overlooked public health problem is noise. Noise pollution is a byproduct of our advanced industrialization and technology. Although research in the area of noise pollution is comparatively new, it is now known to contribute not only to hearing loss but also to stress reactions, irritability, cardiac disease, high blood pressure, and accidents. The public must be educated regarding the potential damage of self-inflicted exposure to noise, such as power boating or loud music, and formulate and implement policies to control the amount of public noise created by aircraft, motor vehicles, and other noise pollutants.

Suggested Activity

Do the following:

- Map areas of noise pollution.

- Describe sources of noise pollution.

- Describe health problems attributable to noise pollution.

- Describe enforcement of regulations related to noise pollution.

- Identify populations disproportionately exposed to noise pollution.

Critical Thinking Questions: What additional discoveries have I made during this activity? What additional information would be helpful to include?

DISEASE VECTORS

Although the emphasis in environmental health has shifted from food contamination and disease vectors to chemical, nuclear, and solid-waste pollution, the control of insects and rodents continues to be a public health problem in many communities in the United States and internationally. It is well known that many diseases are transmitted to human populations by rats and/or various kinds of insects. The role of the mosquito in spreading malaria, yellow fever, dengue fever, West Nile virus, Zika virus, and other infectious diseases is the major incentive for massive mosquito-control programs in swampland areas. Cockroaches and houseflies are common offenders in transmitting gastrointestinal disease through the contamination of food. Insect vectors (agents) transmit disease by sucking the blood of the infected person or animal (host) and transmitting it to another person through deposits in food or through biting. The incidence of tick-borne illnesses has increased dramatically in recent years, causing Lyme disease and Rocky Mountain spotted fever, with symptoms that become chronic, disabling, and sometimes deadly when not identified and treated early.

Suggested Activity

Do the following:

- Map potential at-risk areas for vector-carried disease in the community.
- Map outbreaks of reportable vector-carried diseases.
- Map areas with rat infestation.
- List and date outbreaks of diseases resulting from rat infestation.
- Map insect infestation.
- Describe community health risks associated with the following:
  - Mosquitoes (e.g., West Nile virus and malaria)
  - Houseflies
  - Cockroaches
  - Lice
  - Fleas
  - Ticks (e.g., Lyme disease and Rocky Mountain spotted fever)
  - Bedbugs
  - Biting flies
- Compare community trends in vector infestation with state and national trends.
- Identify populations disproportionately affected by disease-carrying vectors.

Critical Thinking Questions: What additional discoveries have I made during this activity? What additional information would be helpful to include?

The vehicle for control of vector-transmitted disease is entering the sequence of infection at some point to break the chain of infection among host, agent, and environment. This includes prevention and eradication measures, such as the destruction of breeding grounds of insects (drainage of swampland and household sanitation); the extermination of rats that harbor disease-carrying fleas; and the use of insecticides and physical barriers against pests, such as repellents, nets, or screens. The selection of method depends upon the life cycles and natural habitats of the agent and the host. Intervention must occur at the community and the household levels, including health education and inspection programs.

DISASTER AND EMERGENCY PREPAREDNESS

Suggested Activity

Do the following:

- Obtain the local and state disaster plan for the community. Does the community have a trained Community Emergency Response Team?

- Map and date potential emergencies and disasters for the community.

- Describe the cultural capital relative to disaster response in the community.

- How do residents personally prepare for emergencies or disasters?

- Describe the disaster responses to recent emergencies, identifying the following:

    - Local, state, and national involvement

    - Success of the disaster plan in preventing problems

    - Areas for improvement in local and state response capacity

Critical Thinking Questions: What additional discoveries have I made during this activity? What additional information would be helpful to include?

The Federal Emergency Management Agency (FEMA), housed within the U.S. Department of Homeland Security, was established in 1979 to respond to emergencies that overwhelm local and state resources. As noted in Chapter 5, some communities are more at risk for disasters than others, and flooding, hurricanes, tornadoes, and earthquakes can be predicted, expected, monitored, and prepared for in an organized fashion. However, not all natural disasters are predictable; a level of community preparedness to anticipate such disasters is necessary to significantly reduce the consequences. According to *Healthy People 2020*:

> Preparedness involves Government agencies, nongovernmental organizations, the private sector, communities, and individuals working together to improve the Nation's ability to prevent, prepare for, respond to, and recover from a major health incident. (https://www.healthypeople.gov/2020/topics-objectives/topic/preparedness)

An increased emphasis on disaster preparedness has emerged in recent years in response to the Ebola crisis in Liberia and on U.S. soil, as well as to earthquakes and tsunamis in Southeast Asia and Japan, Hurricane Katrina in Louisiana, and the earthquake in Pakistan.

Although not natural disasters, the Oklahoma City bombing in 1995, the World Trade Center terrorist attacks in 1993 and 2001, the anthrax contamination in 2001, and increasing acts of terrorism alerted the nation to a kind of vulnerability previously unimagined. These human-produced disasters are less predictable, and preventing and preparing for them is less straightforward. FEMA, for example, designed a national plan to immunize all healthcare professionals against smallpox after 9/11 and the anthrax threat. One component of this plan was to recruit community/public health nurses as volunteers to National Disaster Medical System (NDMS) nurse response teams to implement a vaccination program.

All disasters have the potential to contaminate air and water; disseminate toxic bacteria; cause massive injury, death, and destruction; and induce pervasive fear, anger, and grief. Therefore, local, state, national, and international disaster-response plans are critical to safeguarding the environment, protecting the population's health, and instilling a sense of control and well-being in the face of overwhelming threat.

CRIME

Suggested Activity

Do the following:

- List the 10 leading crimes in the community.
- Describe changes that have occurred in the kinds and frequency of crimes over the last 10 years.
- Map high-crime areas.
- Describe the presence or the absence of gun violence.
- Describe evidence of gangs and gang activity
- Describe the incidence of reported crimes against women and children.
- Describe the incidence of reported crimes against older people or people with disabilities.
- Identify populations disproportionately affected by crime.

Critical Thinking Questions: What additional discoveries have I made during this activity? What additional information would be helpful to include?

The safety of housing, workplaces, schools, streets, recreational areas, commercial centers, and other public areas requires vigilance and management to promote and protect the health of the public and create a community in which people feel secure. Personal-injury crime constitutes a growing problem that has short-term, and often long-term, physical and psychological implications for the health of the public. Perhaps no other issue so dramatically illustrates the significance of the human environment in the health and well-being of populations. Poverty, unemployment, the availability of firearms and gun violence, drugs, violence, victimization, racism, and sexism all have been correlated with the occurrence of personal-injury crimes (Office of National Drug Control Policy, 2006) as well as a more generalized fear of crime that inhibits healthy community interaction. The incidence of violent crimes against individuals, including murder, rape, robbery, and assault, varies among communities and populations. For some problems, such as domestic violence, sexual assault, and incest, underreporting is common, and accurate statistics at the local level are very difficult to determine; national statistics provide only estimations at the local level. Murder rates, on the other hand, are comparatively accurate. In the 1990s, firearm homicide was the leading cause of death for teenage African-American males (DuRant, Cadenhead, Pendergrast, Slavens, & Linder, 1994). Some 12 years later, young African-American males (ages 15 to 24) had a rate of homicide 3 times that of young Hispanic men and 17 times that of young White men (Kaiser Family Foundation, 2006).

In addition to reducing related morbidity and mortality, *Healthy People 2020* aims for a 10% reduction in the number of firearm-related deaths. Public health efforts in relation to environments conducive to crime include identifying the risk factors and high-risk groups that are correlated with high crime rates. They also include the identification of high-risk behaviors, such as bullying and aggression in elementary and junior high school students, and interventions to teach and model alternative means of conflict resolution.

In addition to having immediate and equal access to qualified protective services, all citizens of a community should be exposed to educational programs to help them avoid and report crimes and to rehabilitate perpetrators of crime. The increase in the prison population in the United States reflects an increase in crimes and the failure of jural-penal institutions, such as law enforcement and the courts, to respond effectively to this crisis. In addition to an aging inmate population, studies have found that as many as 80% of prison inmates have untreated mental illness or substance-abuse problems, yet many penal systems do not have rehabilitation programs in place during incarceration or upon release. The proportion of the prison population that is HIV-positive, has AIDS, or has tuberculosis continues to be much higher than in the general population (Hammett, Harmon, & Rhodes, 2002). The problem of crime and society's response to it is controversial, including, for example, gun control. Public health has a pivotal role to play in prisons and schools as well as the responsibility to inform politicians who establish policy related to crime, personal safety, and the penal system.

ACCIDENTS

Suggested Activity

Do the following:

- List the type, number, and rate of accidents occurring in the community.

- Compare these figures with state and national levels.

- Describe trends over the past 10 years.

- Identify populations affected by each type of accident.

Critical Thinking Questions: What additional discoveries have I made during this activity? What additional information would be helpful to include?

Accidents continue to be a leading cause of death in the nation, especially among young children, teenagers, and older adults. Motor-vehicle accidents are the most common cause of childhood injury. Alcohol use is highly correlated with motor-vehicle accidents, and this knowledge has inspired the now-common driver-education programs in high schools, safe-driver programs for more experienced motorists, laws governing the number of drinks and acceptable blood-alcohol levels, technology to monitor alcohol consumption, and the formation of the organization Mothers Against Drunk Driving (MADD).

The rate of falls resulting in hip fracture in people over age 65 also constitutes a major public health problem, affecting women twice as often as men. Efforts to ensure prompt attention to accident victims, such as volunteer first-aid training, an emergency medical technician program, and adequate emergency transport, minimize the damage as much as possible and any untoward effects, such as fear of falling, sedentary behavior, impaired function, and lower quality of life (*Healthy People 2020*).

The formulation of public policy and governmental regulation to prevent accidents is equally as important. Proper labeling and packaging of poisonous substances, seat-belt laws, and building regulations requiring window guards for young children are all examples of primary prevention policy. Making streets and highways safer for motorists and pedestrians; enforcing domestic and occupational safety codes to avoid accidents at home or in the workplace; and creating safe, protected recreational environments are essential to promote the health of a population.

HOMES AND COMMUNITIES

Suggested Activity

Do the following:

- Describe the range of housing in the community.
- Describe the compliance of housing with state and local regulations for safety, sanitation, and state of repair.
- Identify health risks presented by the condition of local housing.
- Map problems (accidents, fires, and outbreaks of diseases) attributed to substandard housing.
- Identify populations disproportionately affected by substandard housing.

Critical Thinking Questions: What additional discoveries have I made during this activity? What additional information would be helpful to include?

Chapter 5 addressed the quantity, placement, and construction of housing in the community. In the community health assessment, indoor air pollution, adequate heating and sanitation, housing structure, and safety issues, such as exposure to lead-based paint and electrical and fire hazards, are the major concerns (*Healthy People 2020*). Because people spend a large part of their lives in households, the type and condition of housing—including living space, cooking facilities, and privacy—have a profound impact on the health of the population, including the growth and development of children and family interaction. Poor or inappropriately constructed housing may contribute to disease, crime, or safety problems, such as high rates of fires, falls, and other accidents.

Improving the health of a community is highly dependent on the quality of the domiciles in which residents live. Residents must be alerted to the potential hazards of existing housing. Advocacy at the policy level must be accomplished to raise the standard of housing in the community. The kinds of problems encountered in community health practice include lead paint in older housing, radon gas, neglected housing repairs, and safety hazards in the homes of elders as well as young families.

COMMUNITY BUILDINGS

Similar to the private space of the home, the public space of the school, workplace, and other community buildings must have a clean, safe, and acoustically and aesthetically pleasing interior environment. Most communities have codes regulating the capacity of buildings in terms of the number of people who can be there at any one time; the activities that can or cannot take place; the kind and quality of construction or renovation; and the health and safety factors of furnishings and installations, such as plumbing, insulation, carpeting, paint, and wall covering. These regulations on the interior environment are for the protection of the public; breaches of the code require appropriate action. Code violations might include hoarding, poor lighting, sanitation violations in restrooms, not enforcing smoking regulations, asbestos installation, inadequate accommodations for people with disabilities, improper ventilation, and inadequate climate control.

Suggested Activity

Do the following:

- Describe the compliance with local housing regulations.
- Describe the enforcement of occupancy and activities regulation.
- Describe the enforcement of nonsmoking rules.
- Describe the compliance with Occupational Safety and Health Administration (OSHA) standards for occupational safety and health.
- List accidents or outbreaks of disease attributable to breaches of health and safety standards in the workplace or other public buildings.
- Map buildings with health and safety problems.

Critical Thinking Questions: What additional discoveries have I made during this activity? What additional information would be helpful to include?

The workplace is one of the most significant public interiors. The majority of the adult workforce spends at least 8 hours a day, 5 days a week, on the job, where they may be exposed to a variety of health hazards ranging from noise pollution to dangerous chemicals to machinery. Similar to protecting and monitoring the natural environment, solving the problems of the workplace environment is complicated by the economic pressures facing many smaller industries as well as their employees. Even when workers are at risk for serious health problems as a result of some workplace features, they may be reluctant to take unified action if they believe their livelihood will be threatened. Although the protection of workers' health is ultimately in the best interest of the company, employers may be reluctant or even unable to expend the necessary resources. The Occupational Safety and Health Administration (OSHA), an agency in the U.S. Department of Labor, was established to protect workers in such situations.

ENERGY PRODUCTION AND MANAGEMENT

Suggested Activity

Do the following:

- List sources of energy, such as electricity, solar, nuclear, wind, natural gas, coal, oil, wood, and kerosene, used in the community.
- Identify major public sources of energy.
- Identify private sources of energy in the community.
- Describe the adequacy of public power sources.
- Identify wasted energy.
- List health/safety problems derived from major energy sources.
- Describe the methods used to produce energy in the community and the potential safety and health concerns related to the production process(es).

Critical Thinking Questions: What additional discoveries have I made during this activity? What additional information would be helpful to include?

Urbanization, industrialization, and advanced technology require large amounts of energy to create an environment appropriate to the welfare and development of human populations. The conservation of energy is a public health problem that requires community-wide education and governmental regulation. In addition to the potential dangers of nuclear energy already cited, power dams pose the threat of floods, and electricity generation poses the threat of electrocution and electrical fires. The increasing use of wood stoves and kerosene heaters to reduce costly fuel bills also poses the threat of air pollution and fire. Domestic and public management of fuel and energy resources requires an educated public and the enforcement of safety regulations when using these resources.

GLOBAL HEALTH

Suggested Activity

Do the following:

- Identify professionals trained in global health and the detection/management of global disease in the community.
- Identify the nearest CDC Global Disease Detection Regional Center.
- Describe human migration patterns in the community.
- Identify the rates of tuberculosis, HIV/AIDS, or other communicable diseases present in migrants, immigrants, or foreign-born persons.
- Identify the health assessments and immunizations required of migrating persons prior to their entrance into the United States.
- Describe the range of perceptions regarding international and migrating persons/groups in the community.

Critical Thinking Questions: What additional discoveries have I made during this activity? What additional information would be helpful to include?

We live locally, but we are citizens of a larger planet, Earth. *Globalization*—that is, the unification of the people who make up our planet through immigration, migration, and communication—is not a new phenomenon but is now occurring at a staggering speed. Through technological advances in transportation and communication, we can travel great distances in an increasingly shortened timeframe and communicate instantly with almost anyone in the world. Similarly, environmental-health issues and infections know no national boundaries. Global health is defined as follows:

> [A]n area for study, research, and practice that places a priority
> on improving health and achieving equity in health for all people
> worldwide. Global health emphasizes transnational health issues,

determinants, and solutions; involves many disciplines within and beyond the health sciences and promotes interdisciplinary collaboration; and is a synthesis of population-based prevention with individual-level clinical care. (Koplan et al., 2009, p. 1995)

Historically, migration patterns and colonization spread infectious disease, causing much loss of life, such as with the Athenian plague (430 BCE), the Black Death (1347 CE), and measles and smallpox epidemics among Native Americans (17th century). Whether with respect to H1N1, cholera, severe acute respiratory syndrome (SARS), Ebola, or Zika, an awareness of how we affect one another globally was considered sufficiently important for the health of U.S. citizens that it was included as a new topic in *Healthy People 2020*. Furthermore, global health is important because of the unmeasured impact the United States has on the health of other countries where it disposes wastes, such as batteries, computers, and other toxic items and substances. As global citizens, we have a responsibility to know about global health issues and to advocate for a just and good society—one that works to reduce the burden of disease related to poor water quality and quantity, inadequate sanitation, insufficient hygiene, dangerous policies, and inequitable access to global resources.

ENVIRONMENTAL HEALTH HIGHLIGHTS

This section highlights some of the major environmental resources, issues, and problems faced by communities in rural, urban, and global environments. The extent to which the environment is protected from the pollution and contamination that accompany global urbanization is directly related to the sustainability of communities and the success future populations will achieve in obtaining optimum health and welfare. It is clear that for decades, very little thought was given to sustainability of the environment, and society is now paying the price. In a more optimistic vein, although advanced technology has contributed to the problem of environmental pollution, it is equally likely to reduce or eliminate pollution.

Legislation, policy, and economic sanctions are the major tools health workers use to promote healthy environments and to combat environmental problems. Thus, emissions standards for motor vehicles, regulations on dumping of chemical and nondisposable wastes, and bottle-recycling laws will have a greater impact on improving the quality of the environment and reducing the presence of disease, disability, and injuries than any one-on-one patient-care intervention. Many environmental problems require even broader-scale, multicommunity action at the state, national, and global levels. The movement of air and water, for example, carries contaminants across and through many communities, often far away from the origin of contamination and without reference to political boundaries. Effective control seldom can be sufficiently achieved by a local community. For this reason, the federal government has taken a major role in this dimension of public health. The EPA was established in 1970 to coordinate all activities that concern the quality of the environment—the atmosphere, land, and water. It has authority over the states and is responsible for conducting research, providing information, establishing and enforcing standards, and monitoring the quality of the environment.

OSHA was established to develop standards and coordinate safety and health oversight in the workplace. This federal agency regulates policy with regard to tuberculosis control in hospitals and is particularly important for nurses, who are one of the groups most affected by occupationally induced illness. The National Institute for Occupational Safety and Health (NIOSH), housed at the Centers for Disease Control and Prevention (CDC), conducts research on environmental health hazards and recommends federal standards for OSHA and for mine safety. The Agency for Toxic Substances and Disease Registry (ATSDR) was created in 1980. Although it is part of the U.S. Department of Health and Human Services, ATSDR is housed at the CDC and has a comprehensive mission with regard to preventing exposure to hazardous substances. These agencies all have comprehensive websites; two other sites relevant to the environment are Toxnet (National Institutes of Health [NIH], n.d.) and the Toxics Release Inventory (TRI) (U.S. Environmental Protection Agency, n.d.).

POPULATION HEALTH ASSESSMENT

Most people consider themselves members of many different groups. These might include ethnic identifications, age categories, geo-political constituencies, social classes, or religion adherents. In fact, all these classifications have been used at one time or another to categorize people for the purposes of public health intervention, research, and analysis. In Chapter 3, "Learning the Culture and Health of Communities," various bio-statistical measures that describe events at the population level were presented, including birth rates, death rates, and morbidity rates, along with the major kinds of epidemiological studies used to determine risks and probable causes.

Using rates rather than raw numbers enables the comparison of one group with another to discover differences in health status between and among populations. After differences are found, the next step is to ask why they exist. For example, why is the rate of infant mortality different from one community to another? Why is this rate different among racial and ethnic groups or between teenagers and adults? Although the answer is less easy to discover, it is not very different from asking why a patient has a temperature higher or lower than the average body temperature of the human population, 98.6 degrees Fahrenheit.

Life expectancy and health-related quality of life differ among populations within a community. The capacity of a community to eliminate health disparities and to achieve health equity for all is assessed by monitoring rates and trends in those areas in which differences are manifest. *Healthy People 2020* has advanced the national agenda from reducing health disparities to eliminating disparities and attaining health equity for all. *Health equity* is described as follows:

> Health equity entails special efforts to improve the health of those who have experienced social or economic disadvantage. It is a desirable goal/standard that requires 1) a continuous effort focused on elimination of health disparities, including disparities in healthcare and in the living and working conditions that influence health, and 2) a continuous effort to maintain a desired state

of equity after particular health disparities are eliminated.
(*Healthy People 2020*)

Measures to assess the attainment of health for all include tracking of morbidity and mortality rates and chronic health conditions across demographic factors, such as race and ethnicity, gender, sexual identity and orientation, disability status, and geographic location (*Healthy People 2020*). This section contains a discussion of the more commonly collected mortality and morbidity rates and the behaviors that influence them, the risk factors associated with them, and the high-risk groups in which they are found. The categories chosen for organizing these data are not mutually exclusive. AIDS, for example, is an infectious and a chronic disease, and certain health behaviors, such as regular exercise, are equally cogent in school-age children and adults.

Although addressed here as discrete areas, many health problems are interrelated and multidimensional. Interventions to reduce them often must involve biological, behavioral, and environmental factors. For example, problems in behavioral health may accompany disability, the infant-mortality rate is influenced by income level and access to prenatal care, and sexually transmitted infections reflect sexual behavioral patterns that characterize subpopulations, such as sex workers or adolescents.

INFECTIOUS DISEASES

The World Health Organization (WHO), the CDC, and state boards of health monitor infectious and communicable diseases. Certain infectious diseases are mandated as reportable by federal and state law. These may vary among states and are modified as health problems change. In the past, smallpox was reportable until it was eradicated as a public health problem. Some highly infectious diseases (measles and influenza) or diseases that derive from food or water contamination (salmonella and *Giardia*) can result in epidemics. An *epidemic* traditionally is defined as a greater number of cases than expected, found in a particular place at a particular point in time. This flexible definition affords public health authorities considerable latitude in responding to local-level situations. Tracking and controlling epidemics constitute specialized endeavors, and epidemiologists usually are responsible for the initial recommendations for population intervention once their causes and locations are determined. Because community/public health nurses engage in disease surveillance, they may be the first to see these changes and are then responsible for reporting them.

Suggested Activity

Do the following:

- Name the community's five major acute infectious diseases.
- Identify the rates and trends of healthcare-associated infections.
- Compare local rates for the top five infectious diseases with state and national rates.
- Compare current rates of infectious disease with those of the previous 5 and 10 years.
- Note the incidence and prevalence for influenza, HIV/AIDS, sexually transmitted infections (STIs), tuberculosis, and other current disease outbreaks.
- Report epidemics occurring or ongoing in the past year, 5 years, and 10 years.
- Note the incidence of nosocomial infections in local inpatient facilities.
- Identify prevention of infectious disease public health campaigns in this community.
- Identify populations disproportionately affected by infectious disease.

Critical Thinking Questions: What additional discoveries have I made during this activity? What additional information would be helpful to include?

The infectious diseases most prevalent in the United States are influenza and pneumonia, and they disproportionately affect children, elders, and persons who are immunocompromised. Over the past two decades, HIV/AIDS and other STIs have occurred at epidemic rates, with those under age 40, gay and bisexual men,

African-American men and women, and IV-drug abusers disproportionately affected. Most infectious diseases can be prevented through immunization, education, and/or screening.

CHRONIC DISEASES

Valid, reliable, and current data on noninfectious and chronic diseases throughout the world are available through WHO (http://www.who.int/topics/chronic diseases). National data are available through the CDC website on Chronic Disease Prevention and Health Promotion (http://www.cdc.gov/chronicdisease). Noninfectious and chronic diseases increasingly are reported at the community level. These data are frequently available at the state and local community health-department websites. Additionally, many states and regions have cancer registries that provide prevalence, if not incidence, data. Voluntary health organizations, often national in scope (e.g., American Heart Association, American Cancer Society), also are potential sources of morbidity data on noninfectious and chronic diseases, such as cardiovascular disease, cancer, COPD, diabetes, and neuromuscular disease.

The leading causes of death and disability in the United States are coronary heart disease, cancer, and diabetes (CDC, 2010a). Stroke, cancer, and heart disease alone are the cause of more than 50% of annual deaths (Kung, Hoyert, Xu, & Murphy, 2008). Intervention at all three levels of prevention is indicated for chronic diseases, and many are preventable or at least manageable with attention to such risk factors as lack of physical activity, tobacco use, excessive alcohol consumption, and poor nutrition. Because early signs and symptoms often are not recognized, and because health behaviors are related to the most common chronic diseases, intervention strategies at various stages of the disease are critical. With treatment advances, some diseases, such as HIV/AIDS and cancer, have become chronic, suggesting new classifications for some infectious illnesses.

Suggested Activity

Do the following:

- Cite the mortality and morbidity rates pertaining to the following:
    - Asthma
    - Chronic obstructive pulmonary disease (COPD)
    - Alzheimer's disease and other forms of dementia
    - Heart disease
    - Stroke
    - Type 1 and Type 2 diabetes
    - Chronic kidney disease
    - Cancer
    - Arthritis, osteoporosis, and chronic back conditions
- Report the five major noninfectious, chronic diseases reported in the community.
- Report the rates of child and adult obesity in the community.
    - Identify the differences between local rates and state and national levels.
    - Identify the differences between current rates and those of the previous 5 and 10 years.
    - Describe reasons for the trends and differences.
- Describe the primary, secondary, and tertiary health promotion services and programs that exist in the community.
- Identify populations disproportionately affected by chronic disease.

Critical Thinking Questions: What additional discoveries have I made during this activity? What additional information would be helpful to include?

CHRONIC DISABILITY

Suggested Activity

Do the following:

- Cite the rate of people who are physically handicapped or have disabilities in the community.
- Report the disability rate by age and sex.
- Compare these data with state, national, and international rates.
- Compare rates over 5 and 10 years.
- Describe factors that explain trends and differences.
- Identify disproportionately affected populations.
- Describe accommodations that have been made in the community to comply with the Americans with Disabilities Act (ADA).
- List resources available to people with disabilities across their lifespan.

Critical Thinking Questions: What additional discoveries have I made during this activity? What additional information would be helpful to include?

Closely linked to the prevalence of chronic disease is the rate of chronic disability in the community. The increasing age of the American population and concomitant musculoskeletal conditions, including arthritis, osteoporosis, and chronic back pain, are the major causes of disability in the United States. Individuals with disabilities are more likely to be depressed, obese, hypertensive, unemployed, and psychologically distressed.

Healthy People 2020 identifies the following courses of action as three public health goals:

- Improve the conditions of daily life.

- Address the inequitable distribution of resources among people with disabilities and those without disabilities.

■ Expand the knowledge-base awareness about determinants of health for people with disabilities.

Although chronic disabilities may not be reversed, functional ability and quality of life can be enhanced for the disabled population through public action and policies authorizing parking, wheelchair ramps, curb access, public transportation access, special schools, and facilities. These interventions are a component of the public health infrastructure and just as important as clinical management in ensuring quality of life, the ability to function optimally, and productive social relations.

BEHAVIORAL AND MENTAL HEALTH

Surveillance of a community's health status also includes the determination of various types of behavioral-mental health problems. The burden of these kinds of disabilities is profoundly under-recognized in this area (*Healthy People 2020*), yet data are essential for planning appropriate health services, whether ambulatory, residential, or in-patient, and for protective services for victims of abuse and crime. Nearly 25% of U.S. adults experience mental illness each year (National Alliance on Mental Illness, 2013). The suicide rate is a useful indicator of the behavioral/mental health of any population. It is the 11th leading cause of death; approximately 30,000 people commit suicide each year (CDC, 2010a; *Healthy People 2020*; NIH, NIMH, 2007). With improved quality and availability of behavioral-mental health services, people with mental illness and the whole community benefit tremendously. A healthy community offers educational programs on the early identification of mental illness and timely treatment, provides accessible and affordable treatment and support services, and eliminates social stigma, so that individuals affected by mental illness and substance abuse can enjoy satisfying and productive lives, thus improving the well-being of the community as a whole.

Suggested Activity

Do the following:

- Cite incidence, prevalence, mortality, and morbidity rates pertaining to the following behavioral health problems:

    - Severe and persistent mental illnesses (e.g., major depressive disorder, schizophrenia, bipolar disorder)

    - Depression

    - Violence, including domestic violence (child and spouse)

    - Sexual abuse (incest and rape)

    - Suicide

    - Addictions (e.g., alcohol, tobacco, other drugs)

- Compare these figures with state, national, and international levels.

- Compare these figures with those of the previous 5 and 10 years.

- Describe factors explaining the differences.

- Report admission rates for addictive-disorders treatment programs.

- Report discharge rates for alcohol-related illnesses.

- Identify whether homelessness is a problem in the community.

- Identify disproportionately affected populations.

- List services, support groups, and other programs available for people with addictions and/or severe and persistent mental illness.

- List counseling and psychiatric care providers available to people in the community.

- List resources available to people in a mental health crisis.

- Describe how the mental health resources and services are paid for.

Critical Thinking Questions: What additional discoveries have I made during this activity? What additional information would be helpful to include?

MATERNAL, INFANT, AND CHILD HEALTH

Suggested Activity

Do the following:

- Cite the community's maternal-, infant-, and child-health statistics, including the following:
  - The neonatal mortality rate
  - The infant mortality rate
  - The maternal mortality rate
- Compare these figures with those of the previous 5 and 10 years.
- Compare local, state, national, and international rates.
- Cite explanations for trends and differences.
- Report the most common cause of death for preschoolers.
- Report the most common morbidity in preschoolers.
- Identify populations that are disproportionately affected in terms of morbidity and mortality, low birth weight, and preterm births.

Critical Thinking Questions: What additional discoveries have I made during this activity? What additional information would be helpful to include?

Suggested Activity

Do the following:

- Cite the percentage of women receiving prenatal and postnatal care.
- Cite the percentage of preschool-age children immunized.
- Cite the percentage of preschool-age children receiving well-child care.
- Report the rate of teenage pregnancy.
- Report the nutritional status of mothers and preschoolers.
- List resources available to ensure the health and nutrition of lower-income women, infants, and children.
- Identify the percentage of women breastfeeding their infants. Does the community support lactation by providing designated locations for it in public spaces?
- Report the percentage of pregnant mothers who smoke or abuse alcohol or other drugs.
- Identify community resources available that support women's reproductive and sexual health. How accessible are these resources to women of all social and economic groups?
- Identify community resources and programs available that support children's health. How accessible are these to children of all social and economic groups?
- Identify the populations that disproportionately engage in detrimental health behaviors.

Critical Thinking Questions: What additional discoveries have I made during this activity? What additional information would be helpful to include?

Maternal-child health is a designated topic area of *Healthy People 2020*. Significant emphasis is placed on the social and physical determinants of health and the behaviors that promote health, such as early prenatal care, breastfeeding, and smoking and substance-abuse prevention. Traditionally, some of the most commonly used health statistics focus on maternal, infant, and child health as a measure of the well-being of a population. Poverty, access to healthcare, nutrition, social support, age, and the status of women in the community can all affect pregnancy, childbirth, and maternal and infant survival. As such, crude birth rates and mortality and morbidity data for mothers, infants, and children provide a rough, but meaningful, indication of the health status of a population. Most of the risk to infants occurs in the first weeks of life, and mortality rates for this period have implications for improvements in the prenatal and the postpartum environments. The successful outcome of pregnancy and the ability of an infant to survive through the toddler stage provide strong testimony to the availability and accessibility of maternal-, infant-, and child-health services. Therefore, they continue to be used as some of the most significant measures of public health of local, state, national, and international populations.

$$\text{CRUDE BIRTH RATE} = \frac{\text{Total number of live births}}{\text{Total population}} \times 1{,}000$$

$$\text{Neonatal mortality rate} = \frac{\text{Number of deaths under 28 days of age}}{\text{Number of live births}} \times 1{,}000$$

$$\text{Infant mortality rate} = \frac{\text{Number of deaths under 1 year of age}}{\text{Number of live births}} \times 1{,}000$$

$$\text{Maternal mortality rate} = \frac{\text{Number of deaths related to pregnancy and childbirth}}{\text{Number of live births}} \times 10{,}000$$

Morbidity and mortality statistics are most effective in measuring the health of a community when used in conjunction with other kinds of assessment data, such as health-linked behavior. In contrast to illness and disease indicators, health indicators may include, for example, the nutritional status of children as reflected in growth and development statistics, the completion rates of high school students, immunization rates, and well-child care. Federal guidelines recommend that children be immunized by age 3 for diphtheria, pertussis, and tetanus; measles, mumps, and rubella; polio; varicella; hepatitis A; hepatitis B; pneumococcal pneumonia; flu; rotavirus; and haemophilus influenzae type B.

EARLY AND MIDDLE CHILDHOOD HEALTH

Early childhood is birth to age 8; middle childhood overlaps with ages 6 to 12 (*Healthy People 2020*). According to *Healthy People 2020*, these stages of childhood have had little focus in the past, yet they are recognized as including specific tasks that are important to healthy development as well as risk factors, such as asthma, obesity, dental caries/cavities, maltreatment, and developmental and behavioral disorders. The *Healthy People 2020* public health agenda seeks to better understand and plan for the needs of this population, including by encouraging supportive environments, access to high-quality healthcare, and knowledgeable and nurturing families. Schools and recreational facilities are two prime locations for educating children and their families about health promotion as well as disease prevention and management.

Suggested Activity

Do the following:

- Cite leading causes of morbidity and mortality.
- Report nutritional status.
- Cite statistics on vision and hearing screening.
- Report growth and development status.
- Report performance on national achievement tests.

- Cite the proportion of the population that is adequately immunized.
- List the percentage of the population not immunized due to religious or personal beliefs. Describe any outbreaks of childhood diseases that could have been prevented through immunization.
- Cite the proportion of the population receiving routine well-child care.
- Cite the proportion of the population receiving routine dental care.
- Identify healthcare resources (medical and dental) available to children from lower socioeconomic groups.
- Describe community-wide health promotion programs.
- List health conditions that put a child at risk for illness (e.g., obesity and smoking).
- Describe any problems associated with violence, child neglect, and child abuse in this population.
- Report the incidence of childhood depression, mental-health concerns, or suicide in the past 5 years.
- Identify populations disproportionately affected by high morbidity, mortality, or detrimental health behavior.

Critical Thinking Questions: What additional discoveries have I made during this activity? What additional information would be helpful to include?

ADOLESCENT HEALTH

A new topic of *Healthy People 2020* is adolescent health. Included are those persons who are typical adolescents, ages 10 to 19, and young adults, ages 20 to 24, who together make up 20% of the U.S. population (Population Reference Bureau, 2015). Because healthy lifestyle patterns and risky behaviors are established during this time, the goal of *Healthy People 2020* is to "improve the healthy development, health, safety, and well-being of adolescents and young adults" (U.S. Department of Health and Human Services, 2010). Adolescents have been shown to be amenable to socially supported health-promotion programs, such as pregnancy, violence, and delinquency-prevention programs. With increased ethnic diversity in the U.S. population, however, the tailoring of these programs to be culturally informed remains a public health challenge.

Suggested Activity

Do the following:

- Cite leading causes of morbidity and mortality in adolescents.
- Cite nutritional status.
- Cite performance on national achievement tests.
- Report the proportion of the population that is adequately immunized.
- Report the proportion of the population receiving routine healthcare, including sexual healthcare.
- Report the proportion of the population receiving routine dental care.
- List the healthcare resources (medical and dental) available to adolescents from lower socioeconomic groups.
- Report the proportion of the population using alcohol, tobacco, and/or drugs.
- Report the rates and types of violence, neglect, or abuse in the population.
- Identify the "safe zones" that are available for youth (e.g., for lesbian, gay, bisexual, and transgendered—LGBT—youth, runaway youth, and others who are at risk).
- Report the incidence and trends of adolescent depression, mental-health concerns, and suicide in the past 5 years.
- Identify populations disproportionately affected by high morbidity, mortality, or detrimental health behavior.

Critical Thinking Questions: What additional discoveries have I made during this activity? What additional information would be helpful to include?

OLDER ADULT HEALTH

Suggested Activity

Do the following:

- Cite leading causes of morbidity and mortality in the older adult population.

- Report the nutritional status of the older adult population. What percentage of this population has low, normal, and high BMIs?

- Cite the proportion of the older adult population that is adequately immunized.

- Report the proportion of the older adult population receiving routine healthcare.

- Cite the proportion of the older adult population receiving routine dental care.

- Cite the proportion of the older adult population using alcohol, tobacco, or drugs.

- Identify the rate and type of older adult abuse and neglect in the community.

- Report the incidence of older adult suicide in the past 5 years.

- List community resources to support members of the community to remain in their homes as they age. What alternative living arrangements and nursing services exist to assist aging community members as their health and strength decline?

- Identify disproportionately affected populations in terms of high morbidity, mortality, or detrimental health behavior.

Critical Thinking Questions: What additional discoveries have I made during this activity? What additional information would be helpful to include?

It is well known that older adults are the fastest-growing age group, not only in the United States but worldwide (CDC, 2013; Rowland, 2012; WHO, 2015). The increase in life expectancy is a public health success, and it brings opportunities for increased participation of older persons in society. Population-aging also brings an increased risk for chronic disease, such as diabetes, arthritis, dementia, and congestive heart failure, with associated disabilities and social marginalization. Injury prevention is critical for older persons, particularly building healthy environments and lifestyle behaviors to prevent falls—a leading unintentional injury cause of death for older adults (CDC, 2013; WHO, 2015).

With chronic illness often comes an associated need for assistance. Most older adults are cared for by family members or by someone in their own home. With an estimated 1 to 2 million older adults being injured or abused by a caregiver annually (Bonnie & Wallace, 2003), awareness and development of culturally informed caregiver-education and abuse-prevention programs are critical (Institute of Medicine, 2008). It is important to determine what social activities, health-prevention and -promotion programs, and other services are available and accessible to older persons in the community, especially those who live alone. A health assessment should include the identification of hidden populations of elders in the community, such as frail elders living alone and undocumented older persons living with their immigrant children.

Lesbian, Gay, Bisexual, and Transgender (LGBT) Health

The health status of the lesbian, gay, bisexual, and transgender (LGBT) population is a new topic area of *Healthy People 2020* and the national focus for a "call to action" by the U.S. Administration on Aging (CDC, 2013). Identified as a population that suffers high rates of stigma, violence, discrimination, human-rights violations, and health disparities, LGBT populations are more likely to be obese or overweight; use tobacco, alcohol, and other drugs; and, as youth, attempt suicide and be homeless (*Healthy People 2020*). As background to an effective community health assessment, consider the following key LGBT issues identified by *Healthy People 2020*:

■ Prevention of violence and homicide toward the LGBT, especially the transgender, population

- Gathering of nationally representative data on LGBT Americans

- Resiliency of LGBT communities

- LGBT parenting issues throughout the life course

- Elder health and well-being

- Exploration of sexual/gender identity among youth

- Need for an LGBT wellness model

- Recognition of transgender health needs as medically necessary

Suggested Activity

Do the following:

- Cite leading causes of morbidity and mortality in the LGBT population.

- Cite the proportion of the LGBT population receiving routine healthcare, including sexual healthcare.

- Report the proportion of the LGBT population receiving routine dental care.

- Report the proportion of the LGBT population using alcohol, tobacco, or drugs.

- Identify whether violence is a problem in the LGBT population.

- Report the incidence of LGBT depression, mental-health concerns, or suicide in the past 5 years.

Critical Thinking Questions: What additional discoveries have I made during this activity? What additional information would be helpful to include?

OCCUPATIONAL SAFETY AND HEALTH

Suggested Activity

Do the following:

- Describe the predominant employers in the community, the types of industries, and potential occupational health risks inherent in these industries.

- Identify health resources available at occupational sites with the highest risks of injury, and compare them to sites with the lowest risks of injury.

- List the most common health problems found in the adult workforce.

- Report the rate of absenteeism in the adult workforce.

- List the most common reasons cited for absenteeism.

- Report the percentage of the worker population receiving a routine physical examination.

- Report the percentage of the workforce engaging in employer-provided health promotion activities, such as stress-management programs, ergonomic breaks, fitness facilities, and wellness programs.

- Identify occupational groups disproportionately characterized by health problems, absenteeism, and negative health behaviors.

Critical Thinking Questions: What additional discoveries have I made during this activity? What additional information would be helpful to include?

The health of our adult workforce is another measure of the ability of a population to meet the challenges of its environment. The development of health problems or a decrease in performance levels has serious implications for the economy of the community. Many causes of disability are related to the aging of the workforce population, as well as to the work itself and the working conditions, lower-back pain and carpal-tunnel syndrome being two common examples. In addition, alcohol-, tobacco-, and drug-related problems; stress; violence; and abuse often are identified and addressed in work settings that have comprehensive health programs. The workplace is an ideal setting for addressing negative health behaviors and for promoting a culture of healthy behavior.

POPULATION HEALTH BEHAVIORS

Suggested Activity

Do the following:

- Cite the percentage of the population exhibiting the following:
  - Satisfaction with engagement in social activities, programs, and relationships
  - An active exercise program and healthy nutritional habits
  - A smokeless lifestyle
  - Satisfaction with quality of life
- Cite the percentage of the population exhibiting the following detrimental health behaviors:
  - Tobacco smoking
  - Illicit-drug use
  - Excessive alcohol use
  - Overeating or poor eating habits
  - Inadequate physical activity or sedentary lifestyle
  - Living in social isolation
- Indicate the percentage of the population exhibiting detrimental health characteristics, such as hypertension, high cholesterol, and obesity.
- Identify populations disproportionately exhibiting these behaviors.

Critical Thinking Questions: What additional discoveries have I made during this activity? What additional information would be helpful to include?

Health behaviors can be precursors to wellness or illness, often serving to place members of the population in at-risk groups. The CDC has standardized a survey used by all states since 1994 that is reported in the Behavioral Risk Factor Surveillance System, with state-level data provided. Other sources of these data may include the *Healthy People 2020* website and surveys by local organizations on smoking, substance abuse, and sexual behavior. Unhealthy behavior traditionally has been a target for nursing intervention and personal-health services. Its usefulness in community health practice, however, lies equally, if not more, in identifying the disparities among populations and interpreting those disparities in health behavior in relation to community determinants.

The various dimensions of a population-based health assessment presented thus far provide just a sampling of the unlimited range of criteria that can be used to evaluate the health of a population. Depending on the community, certain circumstances or problems may require more detailed information or even different assessment criteria. But it is always preferable to make the best possible use of existing data and to supplement the data with direct observations of a community. Meeting with community members helps you understand their perspectives and can bring the needs of the community to life.

Statistics and other health-status indicators can provide powerful information about the relative health status of a population and convincing evidence about health disparities and the need to take public health action. There are, however, several caveats to consider. As mentioned in Chapter 4, rates must be adjusted or standardized according to demographic characteristics and the size of the community. The morbidity and mortality rates in a small community may be deceptive when compared to those of a large community, and they must be viewed over a longer time sequence to compensate for the small numbers. Most important, the data must be accurate and systematically collected. Death-registry data generally are more reliable than data from birth registries, although one cannot always depend on the accuracy of the recorded cause of death. Certainly, not all births are registered, and not all occurrences of a disease are reported, particularly for stigmatized health problems, such as STIs, psychiatric problems, and alcohol abuse.

HEALTHCARE ORGANIZATION ASSESSMENT

Like education, family, work, recreation, and other human institutions, the pursuit of health has a set of specialized activities, roles, norms, and values in society. *The third component of the community health assessment is an investigation of health and healthcare as a social institution and an evaluation of its capacity to create a healthy community.* All societies have ideological belief and value systems as well as specialized personnel and rituals designed not only to care for the sick (McElroy & Townsend, 2004) but also to promote the health of people in communities.

PREVENTION AND HEALTH PROMOTION

A healthy community meets the goals of *Healthy People 2020*. Thus, *the focus of the public health infrastructure includes economic stability, educational opportunity, a safe and clean environment, robust community institutions, and universal citizen participation.* As a discipline and a profession, public health has endorsed prevention and health promotion as its principal methods for achieving health. Therefore, a health assessment must include an evaluation of the community's infrastructure for prevention as a fundamental aspect of its cultural capital. There are three levels of prevention, each of which corresponds to a set of health programs and personnel that make up the cultural capital for public health promotion:

- **Primary prevention:** The goal of primary prevention is to reduce the occurrence of illness and disability in the community and to increase health and well-being. Primary-prevention strategies for a community's health presuppose a healthy population and ordinarily include clean air, soil, and water; good sanitation; adequate nutrition; and safe physical and social environments in which to live, work, and play. The direct correlation between the standard of living and the health status of a community is a commonly accepted axiom of public health, and many of our most intractable public health problems historically are correlated with poverty (Heymann, Hertzman, Barer, & Evans, 2006; Reagan & Salsberry, 2005). Thus, the effectiveness of primary prevention is measured by the quality of the physical and social environment and community-wide access to health and healthcare, as well as by the traditional mortality (death) and morbidity (illness) statistics. The range of primary-prevention interventions, therefore, could include the creation of urban or community gardens, presentations of early-parenting programs, the installation of traffic lights at busy intersections, the development of culturally informed health-education programming, the institution of culturally informed "walking clubs," nutrition-education programs in primary schools, and sanitary inspections in restaurants.

■ **Secondary prevention:** The goal of secondary prevention is to diagnose and treat public health problems as early as possible and to restore a complete state of health in the shortest possible time. Building community capacity for secondary prevention is accomplished through identifying health risks and problems as well as timely intervention. Primary-care clinics, diabetes-information clinics, disease-screening events, weight-reduction and smoking-cessation programs, river cleanup, driver-safety programs for traffic-law offenders, the razing of dangerous vacant buildings, and shelters for the homeless all qualify as examples of secondary prevention. Secondary prevention presupposes the ability to restore the health and abilities of the community and its residents. Similar to primary-prevention action, secondary-prevention action can be measured by mortality and morbidity rates, but other measures, such as response time of intervention, the proportion of the population screened for specific health risks, and the affordability and accessibility of health and social services, provide additional useful indicators. Police departments, fire departments, neighborhood "quick care" clinics, nurse 24-hour phone triage services, and shelters for victims of domestic violence are examples of cultural capital for secondary prevention.

■ **Tertiary prevention:** The goal of tertiary prevention in public health is to provide the highest quality of life for those persons and segments of the community who have experienced severe trauma or disease, are disabled, or are chronically or terminally ill. Home-care services, hospitals, rehabilitation centers, long-term-care facilities, and hospice are examples of community cultural capital designated for tertiary prevention. With the exception of public hospitals and clinics, which are typically located in major urban centers, the responsibility of public health in tertiary prevention ordinarily is ensuring the safety and supportiveness of tertiary-prevention facilities. This could include safe egress of institutionalized residents in a fire; laws pertaining to patient abuse; regulations governing cleanliness, food services, and staff ratios in long-term-care facilities; and certification of home-health agencies. An outstanding example of tertiary prevention in the United States is the Americans with Disabilities Act, which mandates the provision of access to persons with disabilities.

Finally, although public health departments usually focus on system-level interventions, some kinds of personal-health services qualify as public health–prevention services, because they reduce risk or prevent widespread disease and disability. Such programs not only improve the health of the community but also reduce the costs of expensive hospitalizations and medical care. Well-child care, flu-immunization programs for healthcare workers, home-safety installations for elders, school health services, prenatal clinics, hypertension monitoring, early-detection screening for prostate cancer, and testing for HIV/AIDS are just a few examples.

All three levels of prevention constitute public health action and often are found in a single initiative. Public education for disaster readiness, for example, may be classified as primary prevention. Readiness programs also include immediate and restorative treatment, such as shelters and access to food and potable water (secondary prevention) and the enlistment of hospitals for emergency and acute care of the seriously injured and mental-health programs for those who have lost a family member or suffer from disaster-related post-traumatic stress disorder (PTSD) (tertiary prevention). The integration of programs that support intervention at all three levels of prevention is ideal, not only for optimal outcomes but also for cost-effectiveness.

PUBLIC HEALTH SERVICES: HEALTHCARE INSTITUTIONS

Suggested Activity

Do the following:

- Describe the healthcare institutions responsible for monitoring and promoting the health of the public.

- Describe the process for passing healthcare policies in the community.

- Describe how community health needs are assessed on a regular basis. Include the constituents involved in the process, how the health-improvement plans are developed, and the outcomes measured.

- Identify sources of financing for public health.

- Describe the resources that make up the healthcare institutions in the community, including the following:

    - The number and types of healthcare providers in the community (e.g., nurses, advanced-practice nurses, physicians, specialists, physician assistants)

    - Healthcare organizations (e.g., hospitals, long-term and extended-care agencies, hospice, funeral homes, ambulatory and outpatient care, "quick care" clinics, and home-care agencies)

    - Health-promotion organizations (e.g., fitness clubs, recreation centers, weight and nutrition centers)

    - Complementary and integrative healthcare resources (e.g., herbalists, mindfulness-based stress-reduction programs, Reiki, Ayurveda, healing touch, massage therapy, healing prayer groups, chiropractors, indigenous healers)

- Identify the members of the community prepared to monitor the community's health and provide the necessary interventions.

- Describe the political authority under which the public health system is managed, including officers and boards.

- Identify funding sources for healthcare in the community. Include the roles that public and private health-insurance entities play in healthcare funding.

- Describe the extent to which healthcare facilities are involved in planning for a healthy community.

- Describe the role of the public health system and/or private entities in monitoring and reducing healthcare disparities.

- Describe any public-private partnerships to improve community health and examples of effective partnerships.

- Identify public health programs that exist in the community and their effectiveness for and accessibility to people with the greatest needs.

- List the kinds of new or expanded public health efforts that might be beneficial for the community.

- Describe the function of the Internet, websites, social media, and health apps in the health of the community, and determine the following:

  - The number of homes with dependable Internet access

  - Points of free Wi-Fi access (for example, the local library)

  - The use of the Internet, websites, social media, and health apps in healthcare organizations

Critical Thinking Questions: What additional discoveries have I made during this activity? What additional information would be helpful to include?

According to the U.S. Department of Health and Human Services (1994), the 10 essential services to guide the responsibilities of the public health infrastructure are as follows (CDC, 2010):

- Monitor health status to identify and solve community health problems.

- Diagnose and investigate health problems and health hazards in the community.

- Inform, educate, and empower people about health issues.

- Mobilize community partnerships and action to identify and solve health problems.

- Develop policies and plans that support individual and community health efforts.

- Enforce laws and regulations that protect health and ensure safety.

- Link people to needed personal-health services, and ensure the provision of healthcare when it is otherwise unavailable.

- Ensure a competent public and personal-healthcare workforce.

- Evaluate the effectiveness, accessibility, and quality of personal and population-based health services.

- Research for new insights and innovative solutions to health problems.

Although personal-health services in the United States are considered to be the most sophisticated in the world, the limitations of our public health system are increasingly evidenced by population-health indicators that are inconsistent with the continuing rise in healthcare costs. In its charge to protect and promote the health of communities, managing urgent and chronic threats, our public health system is the foundation for successful population-health outcomes. The three components of the public health infrastructure required to fulfill the essential public health services are as follows (*Healthy People 2020*):

- A capable and qualified workforce

- Up-to-date data and information systems

- Agencies capable of assessing and responding to community health needs

PUBLIC HEALTH WORKFORCE

Public health draws from an interdisciplinary workforce from such fields as medicine, public health, nursing, epidemiology, and sanitation. In 2003, the Quad Council of Public Health Nursing Organizations identified public health nursing competencies for the generalist and specialist that included the following skills:

- Analytic assessment

- Policy development/program planning

- Communication

- Cultural competency

- Community dimensions of practice

- Basic public health sciences

- Financial planning and management

- Leadership and systems thinking

Similarly, in 2010, the Council on Linkages between Academia and Public Health Practice approved core competencies for public health professionals at three levels: entry, management and/or supervisory responsibilities, and senior management and/or leadership (Public Health Foundation, 2011). In 2011, the Quad Council of Public Health Nursing Organizations then updated its competencies to be in alignment with the Council on Linkages between Academia and Public Health Practice (Public Health Foundation, 2014). These competencies are in the same areas as those in the preceding list.

Healthy People 2020 includes objectives to do the following:

- Incorporate the core competencies for public health professionals into job descriptions and performance evaluations.

- Increase continuing-education opportunities based on the competencies.

- Increase the proportion of Council on Education for Public Health (CEPH)–accredited schools of public health and schools of nursing.

- Increase the proportion of four-year colleges and universities and two-year colleges that offer public health or associated programs.

INFORMATION SYSTEMS

An ongoing challenge is to link health-related agencies in such a way that health-information systems can be organized into integrated systems. One effort to systematize information and communication was realized with the adoption by most states of common health-status indicators to gauge community health status and the use of technology to facilitate describing, tracking, and comparing health indicators.

The goals of *Healthy People 2020* include the following:

- Increasing the national data available for all major population groups

- Increasing the proportion of objectives that are tracked at the national level every 3 years

- Accelerating the speed with which national data are released at the end of data collection

- Increasing the number of states recording births and deaths using standard certificates of birth

PUBLIC HEALTH AGENCIES

Not surprisingly, there is great variation among communities in the kind and breadth of their health infrastructures and the services they provide. Also, communities vary with regard to the resources obtainable to address community health problems. One of the great ironies in public health practice is that the communities with the most problems usually have the fewest resources. As discussed in the preceding sections, these health disparities are detectable in the populations and the environments of communities.

Health Departments

In the United States and increasingly throughout the world, the responsibilities for health consist of a complex organization of proprietary (for-profit), voluntary (nonprofit), and public (governmental) agencies that together constitute an increasingly entrepreneurial healthcare system. Most incorporated or geo-politically designated communities—townships, municipalities, and counties—have health departments as part of their government charters. *Health departments* are those organizations ordinarily provided by government statute to monitor and improve the health of the public and the environments in which they live. Typically, they are conterminous with geo-political boundaries and organized in a pyramid of administrative accountability by town or city, county, state, and nation. Historically, physician commissioners have headed health departments, but this structure has changed dramatically within the past few decades as community/public health nurses have been increasingly tapped for these leadership posts.

Health departments vary greatly in their range of responsibilities, but most include environmental and population health services. Usually, they are accountable for the bulk of primary-prevention initiatives: public health education, preparedness, communicable-disease prevention, maternal-child–health promotion, environmental protection, sanitation, the inspection of food and health industries, the regulation of emission standards, and the preparation of vital statistics, to name just a few. Depending on the community, they may be responsible for some secondary- and tertiary-prevention programs, such as control of communicable diseases and direct-care services to underserved populations in the form of primary care centers, chronic disease management, and acute care in public hospitals. Monitoring health disparities and health equity has been added to the responsibilities of more and more health departments across the nation.

Health departments usually are overseen or advised by boards of health. The manner in which board members are selected (appointment or election), the length of their terms in office, and the professional criteria for their selection vary with the local governance structure, as does their role in directing or advising the health department. Their status and position within the wider community and their philosophies on healthcare will strongly influence the contributions of individual members. In small communities, it is not unusual for many of the board members to have little or no background in health sciences or health practice. This provides an opportunity for nurses to educate and advise politicians and other board members about the value of public health services for promoting and sustaining healthy communities and reducing the tax burden on the residents.

Public health departments are increasingly engaging in partnerships with other community entities. In some communities, public-private partnerships forge working relationships to further enhance the health of the community. For example, the Blue Zones initiative has emerged in some communities across the country, with public and private organizations working together to build healthier, health-promoting communities. More information on Blue Zone initiatives can be found at http://www.bluezones.com.

Personal-Healthcare Agencies

Health departments work with local hospitals; extended-care facilities; home-health and ambulatory services, such as clinics; and private practices in ensuring the health of a community. Hospitals, for example, often are viewed as providing only secondary and tertiary services, but hospital blood banks and disaster-preparedness programs constitute a critical component of the community's readiness for emergencies. Hospital records provide important data that can be used by epidemiologists to detect and explain various public health problems. More recently, hospitals have expanded their community responsibilities to play an important role in maintaining the health of uninsured populations through community health–education programs, such as cardiac-health programs, that help individuals extend the years and quality of healthy life. By law, all not-for-profit hospitals are required to provide evidence of the extent and nature of the benefit they provide for their surrounding communities to qualify for tax-exempt status.

Health-Planning Agencies

Most communities have a formal organization officially appointed to coordinate and plan the continued health of the population and environment. In 1946, the federal government launched its first health-planning initiative with the Hill-Burton Hospital Survey and Construction Act. This act provided funds to assist states in financing hospital construction. States were required to formulate a plan for the organization of hospitals and other facilities based on the existing facilities and utilization data. In 1962, federal funding became available for statewide health-planning activities. In 1966, Public Law 89–749, the Comprehensive Health Planning and Public Health Service Amendments, authorized health planning on a state and regional basis. As a result, federally mandated health-planning agencies have been established to ensure that some pressing needs are not ignored while excesses exist in other areas. Such agencies are responsible not only for coordinating and developing local health services but also for including health planning with other kinds of community planning.

PUBLIC HEALTH FINANCING

Traditionally, health departments were supported almost exclusively through state and local public funding from tax revenues, and they provided a limited range of services to residents at minimum or no charge. Now, however, it is not unusual to have at least part of the department's revenue based in fee-for-service activities charged to Medicare and Medicaid funds. The existence of health departments is a clear statement that health is a public responsibility. Unfortunately, because they depend on public funds, health departments are highly sensitive to the vagaries of partisan politics and economic forces. Programs that receive full support in one party's term may be put on the back shelf when another political party takes office. In addition, when fiscal crises arise, public health programs, especially those focusing on primary or secondary prevention, may be sacrificed if they are not "entitlement" programs serving the most vulnerable, such as Medicare or Medicaid.

In the highly entrepreneurial U.S. healthcare system, an assessment of financial resources is very revealing. Facilities derive their revenues from many possible sources, such as private insurers, public insurers, fee-for-service models, charities, and prepaid healthcare plans. The Affordable Care Act aims to make healthcare more affordable to all. Another approach to financing is to look at the resources available to residents, such as self-pay, health insurance, health-maintenance organizations, charities (formal and informal), public assistance, or government insurance (for example, Medicaid and Medicare). In many communities, care of the medically indigent has fallen to the health department and public hospitals. Because all services must be paid by someone, the cost of providing care to noninsured persons ultimately is assumed by the taxpayer or absorbed via higher premiums for private health insurance. In assessing the public health infrastructure, it is important to identify health programs and activities that are publicly supported, without charge or at a nominal charge to qualified residents. These could include school physicals, dental hygiene, immunizations, and prenatal care provided by the health department, plus those services provided by funds raised by voluntary associations or other community groups. The source and method of reimbursement for health services will profoundly affect the distribution, quality, and range of services provided. Despite acclamation for the value of prevention and early detection, unless such activities are reimbursed or supported in some manner, they will continue to be omitted in the range of services provided to communities.

Many uninsured or underinsured individuals and families have no consistent provider of primary care and lack access to primary and secondary services. In this country, patients may not be left to die on the steps of a hospital, so such uninsured individuals and families often rely on healthcare services in the most expensive tertiary venues (emergency departments and hospitals) for conditions that might have been prevented if they had been seen in primary-care clinics. The Affordable Care and Patient Protection Act passed in 2010 is the nation's attempt to increase access to basic healthcare services and rein in escalating healthcare costs. This healthcare reform is a response to the lack of accountability among all three components of the healthcare triangle: patients, providers, and third-party payers. Patients have failed, as a group, to engage in healthier lifestyles; many providers have opportunistically provided unnecessary and excessive services; and insurers have procrastinated in developing reimbursement models that increase the use of preventive services and reduce reliance on expensive acute care. In recent years, the national public health system has taken the lead through Medicare (via the Centers for Medicare and Medicaid Services) by injecting accountability into the system through incentives, such as pay-for-performance formulas, and penalties, such as refusals to reimburse for hospital-acquired conditions and for readmissions to the hospital within 30 days of discharge.

HEALTH VALUES AND BELIEFS

Suggested Activity

Do the following:

- Identify the common beliefs held by local populations about the cause, prevention, and treatment of public health problems.

- Describe common health and healthcare customs within the community.

- List health and healthcare traditions within the community.

- Describe the various opinions of community members about what constitutes a healthy community. Do local residents believe they live in a healthy community? Why or why not?

- Identify three public health interventions that have been well received by the community and three interventions that have generated community conflict.

- Describe local beliefs about illness, palliative care, the dying process, and death.

- Identify the age considered to be a "natural" age at which to die.

- Describe the variations in healthcare values and beliefs present in this community.

Critical Thinking Questions: What additional discoveries have I made during this activity? What additional information would be helpful to include?

The decisions made by health departments and boards of health are heavily influenced by local beliefs and values about public health. Although beliefs about health are not uniformly held or acted upon by all members of a society, it is nevertheless possible to identify a broad range of health ideas, values, and practices that guide and shape the public health infrastructure of a community. Almost all culture groups have theories of etiology or causation that influence behavior related to disease prevention and health promotion. For example, the virus theory of infectious disease explains why individuals contract influenza, but it does not explain why some persons acquire the disease and others do not, even though their exposure was the same. Another example is the belief that childhood immunizations may cause autism, leading some parents to refuse to allow their children to be immunized, despite scientific evidence to the contrary.

The endorsement of public services requires, minimally, that people believe the potential for a public health problem exists and that the problem is amenable to public health intervention. Some members of the community may view violence in schools as a singular, pathological event rather than as an indication of widespread adolescent disenfranchisement or gun laws run amok. Others may view health disparities as just part of the natural order of society rather than as a symptom of an unhealthy and unjust society. Even the most homogenous communities report a lack of agreement on what distinguishes a public health problem from a personal-health problem. The variation in meanings that specific health conditions and behaviors hold for different groups must be considered in planning for the public's health. A lack of understanding between health professionals and the lay public on the definition of a public health problem and the appropriate prevention and treatment can have a profound effect on the success of efforts to build community capacity and ameliorate the problem.

INDIGENOUS, COMPLEMENTARY, AND ALTERNATIVE HEALTH SYSTEMS

When assessing the public health infrastructure of a community, it would be inaccurate to assume that only one health system is operative and that people do not avail themselves of alternatives to the allopathic biomedical system of Western medicine. Rather than making assumptions, it is better simply to ask how people in this community protect their health. How do they make their community a healthier place? The answers to such questions can reveal indigenous local healthcare institutions and the degree to which they are embedded in local culture and connected with other healthcare institutions.

Most populations pursue all the health resources available to them. If, for instance, two distinct systems are in place, it is common for both to be used (Whitaker, 2003). Anthropologists have labeled this "medical pluralism." Given the large populations of ethnically diverse and immigrant groups in many communities, it is incumbent upon community practitioners to know the range of the healthcare infrastructure available within them. Searching the literature to become aware of complementary and alternative health systems that are typically used by the different ethnic and religious groups in your community will provide you with a beginning background to possible health beliefs and questions to ask. This does not, however, translate to what the individual and family members of the community actually do use. Asking individuals is critical, because, by far, the greatest share of personal healthcare in any society takes place in the home, where methods of caring and remedies have passed through families over generations.

Most communities have complementary and alternative healthcare resources and providers who offer healthcare services, such as healing touch, Reiki, herbs, Ayurveda, meditation, yoga, homeopathy, acupuncture, vitamin supplements, and nutrition-based practices. In some communities, these systems are less visible but provide the range of primary, secondary, and tertiary prevention services in a well-organized, internally consistent system that is well known to the community members. Good examples are the *espiritismo* centers found in significant numbers in areas where Cuban and/or Puerto Rican populations reside. These centers usually are located in private homes, where services are provided in the context of group gatherings that have social as well as health functions.

There are several important reasons to acknowledge the presence of complementary and alternative health resources operating in any given community:

- Much can be learned from these traditional modalities, such as the heavy reliance on group and community support as a vehicle for dealing with health problems. The power of group reinforcement, for example, is now being realized in the treatment of substance abuse, diabetes, cancer, obesity, and many other individual and family problems.

- The behavioral norms of subgroups in a community that, at first, may seem odd to outsiders often are rooted in social and/or religious beliefs that have significant local importance in public health. Disregarding or disparaging them can be costly in terms of effectiveness in building community capacity.

- By knowing the logic of complementary and alternative systems, it is possible to place scientific public health practice in a framework that may be more acceptable to community residents. For example, a program for child health and the expansion of prenatal care in a particular ethnic group must take into account norms regarding male and female role fulfillment, age-appropriate sexual behavior, and family structure, as well as the beliefs and practices associated with successful pregnancy and subsequent parenting. Not every client or patient will express the full range of cultural norms regarding pregnancy and childbirth. It is nonetheless important to understand and accept diverse beliefs and practices.

■ The leaders of such complementary and alternative systems are usually charismatic individuals whose local power can be tapped by community practitioners for public health initiatives.

LAYING THE FOUNDATION FOR A HEALTHY COMMUNITY AGENDA

Like the *Healthy People* agendas of 2010 and 2020, a healthy community agenda is a strategic plan, complete with goals, objectives, vision, mission, values, and tactics that permit nurses to get things done in a systematic manner, follow a course of action, and mobilize material and social resources. To be effective, it must be based on knowledge of the community's culture and achieved in partnership with community stakeholders.

CHAPTER 7 OBJECTIVES

- Determine the groundwork necessary to develop a strategic plan for a healthy community.

- Understand the historical and contemporary importance of planning in public health.

- Compare culture-based planning with resource-based and population-based planning.

- Work with community partners to develop a culturally informed healthy community agenda.

- Create an effective constituency for community action grounded in community culture.

- Evaluate the effectiveness of strategic planning for creating healthy and sustainable communities.

THE FUTURE IS NOW

Managing the future is an ethical as well as an operational imperative in community health practice. The public health programs that communities have in place today are based on the predictions and plans that were made 5, 10, or 20 years ago. Similarly, what happens to our children and grandchildren, and the communities in which they will live, depends on the predictions and plans we make today. In the day-to-day work of community practice, however, there are so many issues and concerns that require our attention and effort that it is easy to become distracted from our primary mission: *to promote and sustain the health of our community*. A healthy community agenda is not just a collection of initiatives to resolve particular community problems or issues. It is a thoughtful, comprehensive, and strategic plan, created in partnership with residents, to guide the work we do and the resources we use in shaping the community's future.

The ultimate goal of public health practice is a healthy community. The definitive strategy for public health practice is to work with and through community leaders and groups to enhance community capacity. Finally, you know from previous chapters that a community's health is more than the aggregate of the personal health status of its citizens; it is the capacity of the physical and social community to fulfill the overarching goals of *Healthy People 2020*:

- Attain high-quality, longer lives free of preventable disease, disability, injury, and premature death.

- Achieve health equity, eliminate disparities, and improve the health of all groups.

- Create social and physical environments that promote good health for all.

- Promote quality of life, healthy development, and healthy behaviors across all life stages.

WHY IS PLANNING SO IMPORTANT IN COMMUNITY HEALTH PRACTICE?

Not unlike clinical practice, plans of care are necessary for a healthy community to become a reality. Community/public health practice is necessarily future-oriented. A thoughtful, informed design for the future helps communities effectively manage rather than react to the inevitable changes in the physical and social environments that will take place over the ensuing decades. Health departments in cities and states across the country are giving special consideration, for example, to the future impact of climate change on their communities. The effects of global warming will be especially burdensome for the urban poor, older adults, and those with chronic illness, and they are likely to result in the following:

- Allergies and other respiratory illnesses

- Direct thermal injury from intense heat

- Extreme weather events resulting in injury and exposure to infectious and vector-borne diseases

Hurricane Katrina and the ensuing floods, the tsunamis in Southeast Asia and Japan, the earthquakes in Haiti and Chile, anthrax, 9/11/2001, H1N1, the Ebola crisis, the Zika mosquito-borne virus, and increasing numbers of gun-related incidents all are examples of unpredicted events that require various levels of preparedness. They have sensitized public health departments across the nation to the importance of readiness and have generated the set of objectives for *Healthy People 2020*. These objectives focus on preventing, preparing for, responding to, and recovering from future environmental and social assaults on our communities. Success in responding to and managing such events depends on the extent to which a healthy community agenda uses its cultural capital to create an engaged citizenry, social interconnectedness, government and private-sector collaboration, and a healthcare infrastructure that is prepared to respond.

Dramatic changes in the social and economic context of communities, including industry closures, job losses, housing foreclosures, and population shifts, can also catch communities unaware, with negative results that, in hindsight, might have been avoided.

Iowa has been the destination of a variety of human migrations, including recent migrations from Mexico, Central America, many African nations, and eastern European countries. No one, however, would have predicted a migration of families from Chicago, where urban renewal and gentrification resulted in the razing of high-rise public housing (Keene, Padilla, & Geronimus, 2010). Notwithstanding the decaying condition of the public housing they left, not to mention the associated crime and violence, the displaced Chicagoans lamented the loss of family and friends and the social support they felt in their previous dwellings. Motivated by their desire to pursue a life of "peace and quiet," affordable housing, and better schools for their children, they had great expectations of their new homes in Iowa. Some, however, soon found themselves segregated by a community unprepared to receive the urban, African-American culture they brought with them. The introduction of culturally different young families created a challenge for Iowa-based schoolteachers, healthcare providers, and law-enforcement officials as they tried to interpret and understand the urban lifestyles of this group. They were caught without a community-wide plan for embracing these new members and integrating them into community life. Instead, the existing Iowan community felt "invaded," while the Chicagoans felt "isolated" in a community where occasional gestures of welcome could not compensate for perceptions of racial profiling.

HEALTH PLANNING: AS IT WAS, IS, AND CAN BE

To fully understand the problems and the possibilities of contemporary public health and the significance of cultural information in creating a healthy and sustainable future, it is useful to review the evolution of health planning in the United States.

RESOURCE-BASED PLANNING

Despite the health-planning efforts to promote and protect the health of communities that first appeared in 19th-century England (Gehlbach, 2005), health planning in the United States has focused almost exclusively on the "bricks and mortar" of the healthcare *industry*. Hospitals, visiting-nurse agencies, rehabilitation centers, skilled-nursing facilities, mental-health programs, and so on were established in relation to the demand for services. Utilization experience was reviewed to anticipate and organize health services, with the strategy being to adjust the existing services to the individuals and families who currently used them: If a home-health agency were used to capacity, more nursing staff would be employed or another agency would be opened. Similarly, if a hospital pediatric unit were underutilized, it would be closed or have its staff reduced in number.

Managing demand emphasizes the treatment of health problems rather than the prevention of illness and the promotion of health. In resource-based planning, promoting the health of populations and communities to control cost is not a high priority. Nor is there a great emphasis on reducing disparities or controlling excesses. In response to escalating costs of healthcare, regional models for health-resource management began to appear that attempted to link resources and demands with population size and health needs (White, 1973). Primary healthcare services, for example, which address common but comparatively minor health problems, would be provided in a decentralized model and serve small populations of 1,000 to 25,000. Secondary health facilities (such as community hospitals, extended-care facilities, rehabilitation services, and home healthcare) addressing more serious but common problems would require a population of 25,000 to several hundred thousand to generate a definable demand. Finally, tertiary healthcare would warrant a population of 500,000 to several million to justify the presence of technologically sophisticated and costly services.

Such models for healthcare service delivery based on community-level services inspired the National Health Planning and Resources Development Act of 1974 (Public Law 93–641), which established 205 local health system agencies (HSAs) throughout the United States. Each HSA was accountable for planning the organization of health personnel, facilities, and services in designated districts based on a mandated health-status profile (in most cases, a health-*problem* profile) used to formulate a 5-year health-system plan and an annual implementation plan. Public Law 93–641 was intended to address issues of community prevention and intermediate care, equal access, quality of care, cost, public- and private-sector collaboration, and the maldistribution of services and uncontrolled inflation of hospital costs. The results, however, were disappointing and eventually led to the institution of diagnosis-related groups (DRGs) in 1983 to control the length of hospital stays and, in 2010, the Patient Protection and Affordable Care Act to ensure universal access and to reduce the costs of healthcare.

POPULATION-BASED PLANNING

Although the regional planning efforts of the 1970s did not come to fruition, they paved the way for population-based planning. In the 1970s, a growing sensitivity to consistently at-risk populations shifted attention away from health resources and individuals who use them. By focusing on populations rather than just individual patients, health-planning efforts began to emphasize risk factors and unmet needs rather than illness and resources. Unlike resource-based planning, which emphasizes care for the sick, population-based planning strives to reduce risk through health promotion. The cost-containment strategy consists of primary prevention, health maintenance, early detection, primary care, and the engagement of other social services, including education, recreation, and housing. Based squarely in the science of epidemiology, population-based planning involves four basic steps:

1. Health problems are identified and prioritized, and the population is subdivided according to distinct health needs (for example, women, schoolchildren, elders, homeless people).

2. Risk factors for each problem are identified through a review of the literature, and at-risk or target populations are determined.

3. Interventions needed to reduce or eliminate the problem are formulated.

4. The existing resources are compared with those needed to resolve the problem, and the gaps between them (unmet needs) are designated as essential services that are incorporated in the community health plan.

In population-based planning, we initially ignore existing resources and start with the population's health problems, focusing on what makes people unhealthy or vulnerable. Methods of resolving health problems are not limited to medical intervention or personal health services but include social marketing, policy development, environmental modification, public education, and community awareness. Population-based planning exposes the deficiencies and inequities in healthcare by drawing attention to those groups consistently at risk, often referred to as *vulnerable populations*: women, children, elders living alone without family close by, people living in poverty, those who are homeless, or those who belong to specific ethnic groups.

In population health planning, an increase in the rate of low-birth-weight infants would necessitate a risk-reduction plan beginning with a determination of the affected population and associated risk factors (e.g., economic, genetic, nutritional, occupational, age of mother). This might include family-planning education, smoking cessation, prenatal counseling and monitoring, nutrition programs, and/or workplace-improvement regulation. In resource-based planning, the neonatal intensive care unit would be enlarged to accommodate more infants, and additional specialized staff would be recruited to manage the increasing numbers of low-birth-weight newborns.

By attending to unmet needs instead of demand and utilization, population-based planning holds greater promise for *preventing* rather than *treating* health problems. It is, nevertheless, a deficit model focusing on vulnerable populations and health problems (such as asthma, obesity, coronary heart disease, crime victimization, and traffic accidents). Unhealthy behaviors are treated much like diseases, amenable to such interventions as education, reduction of alcohol consumption, exercise programs, or special diets. Paradoxically, many of these risks are reframed as individual lifestyle *choices* rather than problems embedded in the sociocultural matrix of community life. The population-based approach assumes incorrectly that the public's health could be improved greatly if individuals simply would engage in healthier behaviors.

Because of its problem-specific orientation, the population-based method often yields a categorical approach in which a healthy community agenda is composed of several separately funded and operated programs, such as programs devoted to offering healthcare for women and children, HIV/AIDS, disaster preparedness, lead paint, communicable-disease management, and so forth. Categorical funding has many problems, not least of which is that we often fail to see how health problems are interrelated and could be managed more efficiently and effectively with culturally informed community programs. For example, in attempting to reduce dropout rates among high school students, it becomes quickly evident that poverty, obesity, poor dietary habits, low self-esteem, unsafe driving practices, poor school performance, nonparticipation in sports, unintended pregnancy, substance abuse, drug commerce, and failure to complete high school are highly interrelated and possibly part of the same syndrome.

Categorical programs also have the potential to be divisive, organizing residents around specific health priorities. Pediatricians, parents, and teachers, for instance, will claim that services for children should be the highest priority, because they represent the future of the community. Cardiologists and their patients and families, on the other hand, will argue that cardiovascular disease is a leading cause of death and should be given priority funding. And geriatricians and families will cite the cost benefits of managing the care of older citizens at home to advocate for the prioritization of that population's needs.

CULTURE-BASED PLANNING

Given the history and magnitude of state, regional, and national health planning, why have efforts to control costs ended up costing more and producing less? Why do identified solutions fail to produce the desired outcomes of longer, healthy lives and the elimination of health disparities? And why do health disparities exist in a country that is so rich in resources? At least some of the answers lie, again, in the disinclination to take into account that murky, complex, socioeconomic matrix that makes up a community's culture. The disappointing results of resource-based and population-based plans are not because they were focused on resources or population health but because they did *not* include information about the norms, values, beliefs, and behaviors that compose local culture.

When city health planners decided to close a small, underutilized, formerly religion-affiliated hospital providing limited services, they thought community residents would be better served by a nearby medical center and that resources derived from the closure would be applied to designated initiatives that would improve the health of the community. What the planners did not count on was strong community opposition to the closure of a hospital with a century-long history of serving local residents—as a health facility and as an employer. As such, the hospital in question gleaned sentiment and support from community residents. The dominant ethnic/religious group in the community perceived this action as yet another threat and show of disrespect for its traditions. Champions for retaining the hospital included community members, labor unions, hospital employees, and powerful politicians working on behalf of their constituencies. To the citizens of this community, the closing of the hospital was not just about rational healthcare—in fact, it really was not about healthcare at all. It was about religion, politics, economics, and the social representation of community life. It was about community self-determination. (In the end, the hospital did close and was later reopened as a behavior health center.)

As this case demonstrates, health planning is likely to generate community opposition when the stakeholders have not been part of the process and when the cultural matrix of the problem and the solution has not been considered. Although popular sentiment and modest employment opportunities cannot and should not sustain a costly and ineffective facility, a culturally informed plan could have included converting the hospital to another kind of health facility that would retain employees. Organizers could have enlisted the community stakeholders—for example, hospital workers, political leaders, and religious leaders—early in the planning and perhaps arranged a neighborhood event that celebrated the hospital and its contribution to the community.

A culturally informed plan respects the people who live in the community and makes sense to them. Plans for preventing and treating alcohol abuse in a community where the consumption of alcohol has social and economic value will be different from one designed for a community in which the consumption of alcohol is regarded as deviant behavior. Plans to reduce the rate of adolescent pregnancy will be different in a town where the high school graduation–college–marriage–pregnancy sequence is embedded in the culture, as opposed to one in which pregnancy at a young age is regarded as a normal and welcome event, signaling the transition to womanhood. Likewise, programs for reducing the consumption of high-cholesterol foods may not be welcome in communities where dairy and beef production forms the economic base.

Adolescent obesity constitutes a serious and enduring national problem. In 2011–2012, 20.5% of adolescents ages 12 to 19 were obese. Identified as a national goal in *Healthy People 2000, 2010*, and *2020*, a reduction in the proportion of adolescents who are overweight or obese has been a leading health indicator. Yet after more than two decades, virtually no progress has been made. In addition, as the following statistics indicate, the racial and ethnic disparities in teenage obesity have not only persisted but also broadened to other ethnic groups (Ogden & Carroll, 2014).

Between 1988 and 1994, 2007 and 2008, and 2011 and 2012, trends in the prevalence of obesity in girls changed as follows (*Healthy People 2020*; Ogden, Carroll, Kit, & Flegal, 2014):

- From 8.9% to 14.5% to 20.9% among non-Hispanic White girls

- From 16.3% to 29.2% to 22.7% among non-Hispanic Black girls

- From 13.4% to 17.4% to 21.3% among Hispanic girls

Trends in the prevalence of obesity in boys also changed:

- From 11.6% to 16.7% to 18.3% among non-Hispanic White boys

- From 10.7% to 19.8% to 21.4% among non-Hispanic Black boys

- From 14.1% to 26.8% to 23.9% among Hispanic boys

Using this example to compare planning approaches, resource-based planning would address the burgeoning problem of adolescent obesity in our society by increasing products and services for those seeking treatment. These might include the following:

- Weight-loss clinics with an emphasis on teenagers

- Weight-loss pharmaceutical products marketed to youth

- Special education for providers who work with teenagers

- Increased access to gastric bypass and bariatric surgery

- Self-help groups, books, and programs on weight management that would appeal to teenagers

Population-based planning would identify at-risk groups (non-Hispanic White girls and boys, for example) and try to reduce risk in these populations through prevention. These efforts might include the following:

- High school–based nutrition-education programs

- Regulations requiring the labeling of caloric, carbohydrate, and fat content on foods typically consumed by adolescents

- Working with fast-food restaurants to offer healthy alternatives

- High school–based exercise and fitness programs for nonathletes

- Cooking classes for teens

Interestingly, none of these solutions has yet been effective in stemming the rates of obesity in the population ages 12 to 19.

As with countless other national health problems for which medical treatment and/or lifestyle changes are required (for example, smoking, alcohol and drug consumption, unprotected sex, lack of exercise), the determinants and the solutions are rooted in the cultural context of the communities in which they occur.

How, for example, are dietary practices and food consumption related to local school menus, vending machines, recreation, housing, communication, ethnic traditions and celebrations, the economy, and the beliefs and values about food that guide dietary behavior? Which community institutions have been most effective in addressing obesity (for example, schools, workplaces, places of worship, or health facilities)? How is food consumption linked to school performance, home responsibilities, friendships, and recreation? Basically, when, where, with whom, and why do these teenagers consume food, and what do they eat? Clinical, social, educational, economic, and environmental factors come together at the community level to explain and address the multiple factors influencing diet, nutrition, and, ultimately, health.

Culture-based planning uses strategies from resource-based and population-based planning but expands the epidemiological and problem-based orientation to include cultural inquiry, enabling us to see how problems and solutions are linked to other problems and solutions and to interventions. Although overweight and obese adolescents are a national health problem, solutions and policies generated at the superstructure may not have a predictable outcome at the infrastructure. Well-intended federal and state programs can sink or swim at the local level, where citizens feel influence and exercise power, where resistance or support is most keenly experienced, and where the complex relationship among people, their environment, and social organizations is most reactive. Those who have been involved in comprehensive health planning for a long time can point to national programs for nutrition education, family planning, chemical dependency, prevention, or sanitation that were either redirected or dismantled at the community level, never fulfilling their original intent.

Suggested Activity

Choose a current health problem in your community, and outline resource-based, population-based, and culture-based plans.

- What is the health issue or problem?

- Identify existing community action. Analyze the effectiveness of what is currently being done to address the precursors to and outcomes of this health problem.

- What is the resource-based plan? Describe the healthcare resources that would be required to manage this problem.

- What is the population-based plan? Describe the at-risk populations and the prevention and health-promotion strategies you would use.

- What is the culture-based plan? Describe the health issue or problem within the context of community life and the culture-specific strategies you would use to address it.

DEVELOPING A CULTURALLY INFORMED HEALTHY COMMUNITY AGENDA

In clinical practice, we outline the pathways to desired outcomes through care plans. Using anticipatory guidance, we help individuals and families plan for the future so they will have the resilience and flexibility to manage changes in health and development (for example, bringing home a new baby or preparing for retirement as well as managing a chronic illness or preparing a family for a divorce). But planning is so intrinsic to community practice that it is often difficult to separate it as a distinguishable phase or activity. In community practice, creating and sustaining a healthy community infrastructure cannot be accomplished without intentional, continuous, and long-range planning. Combining accountability for the health of whole communities with personal knowledge of and relationships with residents and organizations, nurses have an unparalleled opportunity to promote healthy communities through long-range planning.

Components of the process necessary to create a healthy community infrastructure identified in *Healthy People 2020* are outlined here. Once again, although they are presented in sequential format, in reality, these components are linked in a dynamic, continuous, and mutually reinforcing process:

- **Overarching goals:** What are the ultimate purposes of our work?

- **Vision, mission, and values:** What are we going to do? Why are we doing this? What are the principles that guide our work?

- **Stakeholders:** What are the existing health-planning structure and organization? How are they linked to other planning organizations? Who are the community individuals currently involved in planning, and which individuals and groups are not at the planning table?

- **Objectives:** What accomplishments will we use to indicate our progress toward a healthy community? What criteria will we use to select objectives? What criteria will we use to prioritize our objectives? How will we measure our objectives?

- **Strategies:** How will we implement our objectives? What is our plan of work? What is our activity plan? What is our strategic plan?

OVERARCHING GOALS

Creating a healthy community is not unlike creating a healthy nation. In *Healthy People 2020*, more than 600 objectives were identified as part of a national agenda for health improvement. Although many of the focus areas and objectives from 2010 were continued in *Healthy People 2020*, 13 new objectives were added to reflect contemporary health and social concerns. Similarly, the myriad objectives included in a healthy community agenda will shift and adjust to accommodate the inevitable changes that take place within the community, the wider society, and the world.

Overarching goals, in contrast, are broader, more enduring, and serve as a framework within which objectives and strategies are selected and implemented.

Building community capacity to meet the overarching goals of *Healthy People 2020* requires the engagement of all citizens and groups in the community's health and welfare, resulting in an empowered community infrastructure that is equipped to manage the relationship between the environment and the population, now and in the future. As culture workers and capacity builders, community/public health nurses are accountable for bringing agencies, groups, and organizations together to design a healthy future for the community.

VISION, MISSION, AND VALUES

An important strength of the *Healthy People* series is that it identifies a vision statement that guides community health planning and anchors the process with a common purpose. For *Healthy People 2020*, it is simply this: "A society in which all people live long, healthy lives." This statement has the power to bring varied and often disparate groups to a common goal. Although there may be disagreement about the strategies and activities composing a healthy community agenda, each one ultimately must contribute to the vision.

A *vision statement* expresses what or who you are and why you are engaged in this process. In general, the simpler the vision, the better. A *mission statement*, on the other hand, describes what you are here to do and what distinguishes you from others with a similar mission. The mission of a college of nursing may be to prepare the next generation of leaders in the profession. The mission of a hospital may be to provide patient-centered acute care. The mission of a restaurant may be to serve fresh and wholesome food to discerning customers. Usually, mission statements are longer than vision statements and are more explicit. For example, the mission statement for *Healthy People 2020* is to strive to do the following:

- Identify nationwide health-improvement priorities.

- Increase public awareness and understanding of the determinants of health, disease, and disability and the opportunities for progress.

- Provide measurable objectives and goals that are applicable at the national, state, and local levels.

- Engage multiple sectors to take action to strengthen policies and improve practices that are driven by the best available evidence and knowledge.

- Identify critical research, evaluation, and data-collection needs.

A *value statement* identifies the principles by which a mission is accomplished. An example of a value statement could be: "All people have the right to health and healthcare." This statement lets everyone know that this value cannot be violated in the pursuit of the mission. It is not an empirical statement but rather an ethical/philosophical statement grounded in societal and professional norms. Although it is important to clarify and endorse values to guide the planning process, ultimately, the true values or norms of a society are exposed through actual behaviors. The realities of widespread health disparities and disenfranchisement of whole sectors of community residents probably reveal the most about our social values regarding who is entitled to health and who is not. An objective appraisal of our highly entrepreneurial healthcare system might indicate that the true driving value of contemporary healthcare is that sophisticated and expensive medical procedures will be reserved only for those who have the ability to pay; however, such a statement would be inconsistent with the normative values endorsed by our society. During the planning process, it is useful to acknowledge the range of values that may be revealed to identify some shared value as a starting point. Although *Healthy People 2020* does not have a specific value statement, its guiding values are evident in its vision, mission, and overarching goals: health equity, good science, high quality, equal access, public awareness, prevention, community engagement, and interdisciplinary action.

Suggested Activity

Do the following:

- Write a vision statement for your community action plan or project.

- Write a mission statement for your community action plan or project.

- List the values that guide your community action plan or project.

- List the strategies that will promote sustainability of the community action plan, as appropriate.

COMMUNITY PARTNERS, STAKEHOLDERS, AND COMMUNITY ACTION

In most localities, public and private healthcare organizations (e.g., the New York City Department of Health and Mental Hygiene, Heartland Alliance, the Lions Club, Beta Zeta Chapter of Sigma Theta Tau International, and the Atlanta Heart Association) already are involved at some level in health planning. Using community culture inquiry data, the first step is to identify the organizations and individuals currently engaged in planning for the health of a community. As described in Chapter 5, "Discovering the Culture of Your Community," and Chapter 6, "Determining the Health of Your Community," the characteristics of the planning infrastructure and its membership will vary with the community, reflecting local values and social organization. Ideally, the community health-planning infrastructure will communicate with other planning groups (e.g., education, arts and culture, faith organizations, housing, and transportation). To ensure the most cost-conscious and effective planning, coordination with health-planning organizations in neighboring communities or at the municipal, county, state, and national levels is highly desirable.

Citizen participation is not new in health planning. From the Hill-Burton Act in 1946 to the mandated citizen majority in the 1974 Health Planning Act, community partnerships have been a hallmark of public health practice. Although the early years of mandated citizen involvement led to some disillusionment regarding the role and function of citizens (Steckler & Herzog, 1979), contemporary provider groups and organizations ordinarily welcome the presence of community residents who not only will interpret the community and its culture for others but also will facilitate the implementation of health plans. As we know, however, a community citizenry is not necessarily of one mind. Although planning goals come from an assessment of community needs, they are modified and prioritized in relation to the availability of resources and competing community interests. It is normal for the goal-setting process to be sometimes contentious and politicized in the competition for limited resources. It also is normal for citizen representatives to be as self-interested as any other board members and to disagree with other self-interested citizens, perhaps more than they disagree with the professionals on the board. Finally, although community partnerships are essential for a successful community health practice, they are not a substitute for the systematic assessment and analysis of the community culture.

The selection of community stakeholders and partners to serve on a board or coalition must be grounded in cultural knowledge about who they are in the community; to whom they are related; their political, religious, and occupational affiliations; their public interests; and their potential conflicts of interest.

The health of a community is the shared responsibility of all its residents and institutions. One measure of successful planning is the extent to which it provides the opportunity for the voices of all community members to be heard through active involvement in subcommittees, consultations, or public hearings. Health disparities and quality-of-life issues, in particular, mandate the engagement of multiple sectors of community life, such as education, religion, government, the economy, and recreation. In culture-based planning, local stakeholders become invested not only in solving current problems but also in understanding the culture of their community, identifying and prioritizing health needs, and creating a healthy community agenda for the future.

During the 1970s, a community-service group from the United States was working with villagers on a Caribbean island. They noticed a large, two-story building housing older and disabled villagers. Because the building had only one staircase, people with disabilities living on the second floor were unable to access the outdoors. To address this problem, the U.S. group—in partnership with officials from key island organizations—planned and built a wheelchair-accessible ramp from the second floor to the yard surrounding the building. This intervention was developed through consultation with key community members and intended to enhance the lives of the confined residents, but in reality, it permitted confused people with disabilities to go down the ramp alone and become lost in the surrounding rainforest and even drown at sea. Although the intent to provide access to the outdoors was a good and culturally appropriate effort, with only two caregivers to assist more than 50 older and disabled residents, the results were disastrous. A systematic community-cultural inquiry and community health assessment in addition to the consultation with local residents and the caregivers might have predicted and prevented the untoward outcomes of this well-intended plan.

OBJECTIVES

Objectives refer to the specific measurable or documented targets used to trace the progress necessary to reach goals.

Identifying Objectives

Our community health assessment from Chapter 6 revealed the explicit objectives we want to include in our healthy community agenda. As described in the Community Tool Box (KU Workgroup for Community Health and Development, 2015), the objectives identified in *Healthy People 2020* tell us how we are doing in achieving the nationwide agenda for health. They are specific and calculable milestones to be accomplished at a certain level and within a certain timeframe. To be included in *Healthy People 2020*, objectives must:

- Be prevention-oriented.

- Drive action that will work toward the achievement of the proposed targets.

- Be useful and reflect issues of national importance.

- Be measurable and address a range of issues.

- Be continuous and comparable.

- Be supported by the best available scientific evidence.

- Address population disparities.

- Be valid, reliable, and drawn from nationally representative data.

No single *Healthy People 2020* objective will apply to all communities, nor will all objectives apply to any one community. Similarly, a healthy community agenda is composed of many objectives, some of which will apply only to certain sectors of the community but, in concert, will improve the health of the whole community. Although it is likely that many community objectives will be similar to those in *Healthy People 2020* and may use the same measures for progress, the identification of objectives and strategies begins with the community. The objective to improve public high school completion rates, for example, may apply to many communities, but the causes of the problem and the strategies for the solution will vary significantly from community to community.

One of the objectives of *Healthy People 2010* was to eliminate ethnic disparities in high school completion rates. Dropping out of school is associated with deferred employment, poverty, and poor health. The target of 90% set for this objective was consistent with the national education goals to increase the high school graduation rate of all ethnic groups to at least 90%. In 1996, only 62% of Hispanic/Latino and 83% of African-American youth, ages 18 to 24, had completed high school, compared to 92% for White, non-Hispanic youth (*Healthy People 2010*).

In *Healthy People 2020*, the health and social problems of teenagers and their impact on the neighborhoods where they live were considered sufficiently important to create a new topic area for adolescent health, with 11 objectives and 24 measures. The 2010 high school completion rate objective, which was not achieved, was modified in 2020 as follows: "Increase the proportion of students who graduate with a regular diploma four years after starting ninth grade." A target of 82.4% was established, using a baseline of a 74.9% average graduation rate for public school students graduating with a regular diploma in 2007–2008.

In one community, low high school completion rates may reflect the need for teenagers to economically assist their families by entering the workforce while they are still in high school. In another community, high school completion rates may be linked to a high rate of teenage pregnancy. In still another, they may be associated with drug use and commerce. If some residents remain unconvinced of the importance of a problem, its solution will require a different strategy than if the problem has uniform community support. For example, in some communities, it may be inappropriate to focus on reducing the rate of adolescent pregnancy to achieve the high school completion rate goal of 82.4%. The optimal life stage in which to become pregnant is guided by cultural tradition, religious canons, and socioeconomic factors. In communities that are culturally comfortable with teen pregnancy, a more effective solution for improving high school completion rates would be to remove the barriers that prevent teen mothers from completing high school.

Prioritizing Objectives

A culturally informed approach, using the community's timeframe, will create an effective and realistic schedule for pursuing a healthy community agenda. The overarching goals of the healthy community agenda provide a useful set of criteria by which to prioritize objectives (*Healthy People 2020*):

- What is the extent of risk to the entire community if the problem is unresolved?

- Is there a need to resolve one problem before another problem can be addressed?

- To what extent will the solution of one problem solve many other problems?

Our cultural knowledge of the community helps us more accurately forecast the determination of the relative importance and timing of initiatives. *Forecasting* is the process of predicting what would happen if one objective were selected to precede another as well as what would happen if nothing were done about the problem. For example, given the close relationship between education and personal-health behavior, mental health, family dysfunction, crime, unemployment, substance abuse, and domestic violence, an extraordinarily compelling case can be made for increasing the rates of high school completion.

Finally, the reconciliation of professionally identified needs and community-identified demands is an important part of priority setting. Residents may believe, for example, that adolescent sexuality is a serious problem that must be addressed in the context of high school completion. In contrast, the provider community may be less concerned with the relatively few occurrences of adolescent pregnancy compared with documented, widespread cigarette smoking by adolescents. The goal is to bring the community perspective and the provider perspective together in a culturally informed, prioritized plan for adolescent health.

Measuring Objectives

An effective healthy community agenda requires not only prioritized objectives but also indicators that you have achieved them. Once the objectives have been prioritized, they must be translated into measurable outcomes, or targets, that will demonstrate the attainment of a goal. The objective to improve public high school completion rates is data-driven (from an analysis of education statistics) and value-driven (from the principles of social justice and equity). It must be stated, however, in a way that will make progress measurable. What specific behaviors or events are desired? The objective would then be phrased in behavioral or measurable terms. For example, the target rate set for 4-year high school completion in *Healthy People 2020* is 84.2%.

In addition to stating the target outcome, it is necessary to state the timeframe within which the outcome is expected. This will depend on the nature and extent of the problem, the resources available, and the culture of the community. In some communities, it may be realistic to say that improvement in public high school completion rates will be 95% in 4 years, while others may require a longer period to reach 80%. Using interim benchmarks to revisit outcomes on an annual basis, the timeframe must be consistent with the length of time necessary to measure the effects. Increasing the rate of high school completion, for example, may take much longer than improving teenage-driving safety, which is more amenable to regulation and policy. Successful accomplishment of interim benchmarks or short-term goals is helpful in providing encouragement to planners and stakeholders. It is important, however, that long-term, truly consequential goals representing real progress in improving health and reducing disparities not be forgotten in the wake of short-term success.

STRATEGY

The notion of *strategy* captures what we understand to be the most effective way of accomplishing our objectives and overarching goals in a particular place at a particular time in the context of a particular culture. Strategic planning for a healthy community agenda is covered in detail in the next chapter. For now, the most important thing to know is that formulating the most appropriate and effective long-range strategy for creating a healthy community requires looking deeply into its culture—not only the characteristics of the population but the physical and social cultures as well. Only through this penetrating analysis of the community will the culture-specific facilitators and barriers in a long-range strategy be revealed. It is not enough to simply go through the process identifying the overarching goals, vision, mission, and values and the objectives; to make the plan truly strategic, the process must answer each of the planning questions *with reference to the particular community and its special place in the universe.*

For example, to make a strategy come alive in La Crosse, Wisconsin, those generalized questions that precede the formulation of a strategic plan must be asked *specifically* about and for La Crosse:

- What is the ultimate purpose of our work in La Crosse?

- What are we going to do in La Crosse?

■ Why are we doing this in La Crosse?

■ Why are we doing this *now* in La Crosse?

■ What are the principles that guide the culture of La Crosse and, ultimately, our work?

■ How is health planning carried out now in La Crosse? Who is *not* at that table?

■ Who are the La Crosse stakeholders?

■ What accomplishment will we use in La Crosse to indicate our progress?

There is simply no other way to identify the cultural capital that will facilitate the plan and no other way to identify the cultural barriers to implementation—both of which make up the strategic plan. While two communities may manifest the same problem, they are likely to articulate very different plans for its solution and very different strategies to get there.

Public High School Completion: Contextual Analysis

Objective: Improve High School Completion Rates	Population: Adolescents	Target Population: Adolescents at Risk
Physical environment: space and time	Where do adolescents live (which neighborhoods)?	Where do target teens live (which neighborhoods)?
	Where do teenagers spend their time?	Where do target teens spend their time?
	How do teenagers organize their day?	How do target teens spend their day?
	Where do they recreate?	Where do they recreate?

The population	How many adolescents are in the community?	How many at-risk adolescents are in the community?
	What are the demographics?	What are the demographics?
	Sex	Sex
	Religion	Religion
	Ethnicity	Ethnicity
	Class	Class
	Residence	Residence
	Grammar school	Grammar school
	Housing	Housing
	Economics	Economics

From this cultural information about our target group in the community context, we begin to determine how cultural capital, such as local institutions, individuals, and groups, can be identified and mobilized to address the problem. If young people have to leave school to help support their families, the strategies for improving high school completion rates will be very different from strategies used in a community in which a high dropout rate is attributed to the use and sale of illicit drugs. Depending on the context of the problem, there will be different cultural capital, different stakeholders, different timeframes, and different strategies. This informs how one analyzes the appropriateness of best practices and/or evidence-based programming to address the issue. Successful community advocacy and partnership are related directly to (a) how well community cultural information is collected, organized, and applied; and (b) the effectiveness of the relationships established with community residents and groups.

BUILDING A CONSTITUENCY FOR CULTURE-BASED ACTION: DO WE NEED IT? WHO SHOULD BE ON IT?

Traditionally, nurses have derived their influence through their delivery of various means of "nursing care." The counsel, care, and comfort they provide to patients and their families—continuously and in times of crisis—are powerful means for establishing and securing relationships. To build a community-wide base of support, however, *the authority and profound influence of nurses must reach beyond the private domain of home, family, and acute care setting and into the public arena.* Community constituencies are built by knowing and being known by the key citizens and organizations in all their various dimensions. Issues of health and illness potentially affect every member of a community, either directly or indirectly, and community/public health nurses are experts on how people can stay well and manage health problems. That expertise has a powerful influence on community residents. As prominent members of the community whose mission is highly valued, community/public health nurses have access to influential members of their communities. In recent history, most nurses have been unaware of the magnitude of their influence and are unaccustomed to using their influence, even though the frequency and nature of their contact with all sectors of the population would be the envy of any legislator. Politicians, on the other hand, are acutely aware of the influence nurses command as individuals and as professionals who have generated the admiration, respect, and confidence of community residents. Legislators and other public officials are eager to make the acquaintance of nurses and to work with them on a variety of health and social issues.

Now is the time for nurses to recognize the power of influence and to use it for the betterment of the community, in the spirit of Lillian Wald's leveraging her influence for the health of immigrant families living in the New York tenement buildings.

Identifying and making personal contact with influential residents in the community is essential for building community relations and is probably the most fundamental skill of successful community/public health nursing practice. Even in the early stages of community assessment, it is possible to recognize potential constituents and identify your potential importance to them—for example, suggesting to a young television reporter that she will be first on your list of people to call with an interesting story about the health of the community, or letting a political official know that your office would be happy to provide her health aide with the necessary statistics to use in her next speech. Or it could be as simple as establishing a personal connection—for example, graduating from the same college, playing bridge, or sharing Swedish ancestry. Begin to build your network of influential persons with whom you can communicate regarding community health issues. Look for ways to build relationships at a community or professional meeting. When you meet an influential person, ask to be introduced to other influential people before the meeting is over. Additionally, it is important to remember that your role in the community renders you an influential person who will be called upon for your expertise.

Finally, one of the most important vehicles for connecting community practitioners with influential decision-makers is a community advisory board. The choice of whom to invite to serve on your advisory board should derive directly from the roles and positions of these individuals in the community and their capacity to assist in building a power base for health planning. The real value of such boards is not widespread citizen participation or even representation; those goals can be achieved in a number of other ways. Rather, community advisory boards should extend the influence of community/public health nurses into social and economic arenas. Typically, board members sit on several community boards, potentially expanding your influence and connection. Of course, it is incumbent on community/public health nurses to give back to the community by volunteering to serve on advisory boards in the many diverse sectors of the community—the city finance committee, an urban-planning task force, or the board of education.

Suggested Activity

Do the following:

- From your community assessment, list six individuals or groups that would be valuable as members of your community constituency, your rationale for choosing each person or group, and what strategies you will use to meet with and recruit them.

Who	Why	How

Recruiting and engaging stakeholders in formulating goals, objectives, and strategies lay the groundwork for a citizen action that is culturally informed and community-specific. Grounded in the overarching goals of *Healthy People 2020*, planning in partnership is essential for creating a better future.

LEADING CULTURALLY INFORMED COMMUNITY ACTION

Making the broad, far-reaching changes that will achieve health equity, eliminate disparities, create healthy environments, and promote quality of life for all requires stakeholders coming together for system-level action. This chapter works through the complex process of leading change and building community capacity by putting a culturally informed healthy community agenda into action to expand community capacity.

CHAPTER 8 OBJECTIVES

- Distinguish between the conflict and the consensus models of public health action, and use them appropriately.

- Identify the special challenges of communities as clients.

- Apply the principles for building effective coalitions.

- Distinguish between primary and secondary target groups in mobilizing community action.

- Distinguish between a conservative and a culturally preservative action plan.

- Understand the principles of a culturally informed public health case statement.

BUILDING CAPACITY THROUGH CITIZEN ENGAGEMENT

Building capacity for community action and change is not just about creating equitable partnerships with community residents and groups to solve specific health problems. Rather, it is a perpetual set of activities that begins with assembling and maintaining an inventory of the community's cultural capital and continues with engaging individuals and organizations in building community capacity (McKay & Hewlett, 2009). Just as clinicians are responsible for collecting, applying, and communicating comprehensive knowledge about their patients, community/public health practitioners are the custodians of knowledge about the community. We are accountable for ensuring that cultural information is collected, organized, and then deployed to enhance the public's health. Creating a sustainable, healthy community equipped to accommodate challenges and opportunities and to manage problems as they occur requires culturally informed community engagement and leadership.

GUIDING CHANGE: A CULTURALLY PRESERVATIVE APPROACH

Change cannot be considered out of context. The nature, extent, and speed of planned change depend on the problems being addressed and the cultural milieu in which they occur. The mandate in public health practice is not change for the sake of change but rather change for the purpose of ensuring and promoting the health of the public. This may or may not require major alterations in community life, and before planners determine how change should be accomplished, they must first determine whether change is necessary. The goal of culture-based planning is not to accelerate change nor to restrain it; instead, it is to manage it with minimal upheaval and cost while providing significant benefit to the community. A major challenge for contemporary communities is to generate a community health plan that has sufficient flexibility as well as durability to survive in a rapidly changing world.

Effective capacity building is grounded in an understanding and appreciation of local traditions. This *culturally preservative* approach to civic action is not to be confused with an incremental or conservative approach. The preservative approach is based on the notion that it is possible to accomplish profound and often very rapid change with minimal disruption by casting change in the context of community culture. The effectiveness of health action is related directly to our familiarity with the logic of local customs and behavior and how community life is organized. On first entering a community, our attention typically is drawn to its problems and limitations. As we come to know the culture of our community client better, however, many of the features of community life that initially appear to be weaknesses may, in fact, turn out to be assets and strengths. Behavior that seems almost self-defeating becomes intelligible when viewed within the cultural framework of community life.

> To promote quality of life for rural older adults, the county nurse arranged to pick up their medications twice a week at a less-expensive national-chain pharmacy located in a city where she resided. To her surprise, the older adults preferred to continue purchasing their medications at their local pharmacy, where they paid significantly more. At first, this behavior appeared to be irrational. A cultural inquiry of the community, however, revealed many features about this rural community that were not immediately obvious. The pharmacy was a family-owned business that had served the community for generations. The current pharmacist and her husband lived in the neighborhood and attended the same church as many of their customers. Their children attended the local public school, where the husband taught fifth grade. The pharmacy sponsored many community events and organizations, including a Little League baseball team and a winning high school girls' basketball team. Without the advantages of a volume business, the pharmacy charged residents more than they would pay through a national pharmacy chain. Yet to not patronize this local business would have offended a well-known family and constituted a serious breach of community culture.

Community residents understand these subtleties and explain the value of having a pharmacist who knows you, who is willing to get up in the middle of the night when someone needs medication right away, and who will give you a month or two to pay your bill, if necessary. The residents of this community have a relationship with their pharmacist. They are committed to her, and she to them. Disregarding the patterns and institutions that have been established over decades would seriously jeopardize the building of relationships for community collaboration. Rather than focusing exclusively on the shortcomings of community life or attempting to organize what already is organized, *successful community action must begin with respect for local values and traditions.* We must be willing to suspend our judgment until we build the relationships with residents that permit us to discover the internal logic of our community client.

MODELS FOR COMMUNITY ACTION

Trying to get things done to enhance the current and future health of communities can be a complex process. We may be challenged by unanticipated conflict and controversy in working with communities we assumed to be unified in purpose but who are, in fact, composed of individuals and groups with divergent preferences and priorities. We have known for more than a half century that opposing factions can be found in even the tiniest villages (Wellin, 1955), but it was not until the introduction of ethnography into public health science that the realities of communities as unwieldy, complicated, and heterogeneous matrices were revealed (Bibeau, 1997; Drevdahl, 2002; Skemp Kelley, 2005a,b,c; Skemp, Maas, & Umbarger-Mackey, 2014). Nevertheless, the image of communities as composed of like-minded citizens united by a common purpose for collective action has continued to permeate public health theory and practice (Bibeau, 1997; Clark, 2007; Davis, 2000; Minkler, 2005; Rosen, 1954).

These different perceptions reflect fundamentally different theories about the nature of communities. One is that communities are held together by a common ideology and value system. The other is that communities are held together by the diversity of values and goals and the capacity of members to meet each other's needs. Applying these two paradigms to the familiar example of a college or a university, one interpretation is that students, faculty, and administrators are held together by their shared academic values; another interpretation is that students, faculty, and administrators have different values and goals and are held together through a complex exchange of knowledge, money, and services. Like all communities, some things are shared by all the members of the university community, such as pride in a winning basketball team, while others are not, such as the need to increase the cost of tuition.

In community/public health nursing practice, these two theories about what holds communities together have generated two different models for leading change:

- **The consensus model:** The long-standing consensus model assumes communities are defined by a shared set of core values around which members can be organized to reach agreement and to achieve common goals (Minkler, 2005). Change is centered on achieving community-wide collaboration, including endorsement by the existing power structure. The methods typically used in the consensus model are enhancing communication, offering moral and rational persuasion, and building rapport. This definition has underpinned community health action and promoted strategies for change, such as values clarification, public education, exchange of ideas, and opportunities for relationship building and communication.

- **The conflict model:** The conflict model, proposed by the founder of modern community organizing, Saul Alinsky (1971), assumes the existence of inherent conflicts and competition in all human groups, including communities. It is based on the belief that self-interest as well as the common good guide the behavior of most people. Rather than stressing the commonalities among community members, the conflict model takes into account status differences, rival affiliations, and power relationships. In the conflict model, sweeping change in a community is likely to require realigning power rather than working with the existing power structure. Acknowledging vested interests, multiple community roles, conflicting values, and power struggles, the existing decision-making process is altered through social affiliations and political action. In a factory, for example, management needs the human labor provided by workers, and workers need the income provided by management. In this exchange, both parties give something and get something. Change, therefore, can take place if one of the parties withholds what the other wants.

The conflict model does not always involve resistance; it often means building bridges between groups that normally have little contact with one another so that members can get to know each other. When this happens, stereotypes often break down, and people begin to bring their reference groups together in a spirit of cooperation. Once again, these bridges are not necessarily predicated on shared values, goodwill, or humanitarian interests; rather, they depend on the notion that each group has something the other needs or wants. By understanding the nature of self-interest, relationships can be facilitated between and among people who can accomplish their own goals while promoting the health of the public. In other words, the way to deal with vested interests is to understand them and to apply them. Rather than be put off by what may be construed as greed and opportunism, self-interest can be the pillar for formulating a strategy that will accomplish a healthy community agenda.

> In an eastern city, parents requested that the city council designate certain blocks as "play" streets so they could open fire hydrants on hot summer days. Some councilors endorsed this endeavor, because they believed the safety and quality of life for children was important. Others had little interest in the project but supported it because their fellow councilors had supported their causes in the past. Together, their backing resulted in a sufficiently broad base of community support to counter opposition from residents who felt inconvenienced by the closing of streets.

At first, the conflict model may appear to be socially manipulative, but the fact that people vary in their commitments to what we may define as a worthy cause is simply a reflection of different priorities. Some citizens will support programs for older adults but be indifferent to people with disabilities; others will support adolescent programs but disregard the homeless. In the conflict model, whether people give money to support a community health initiative because they believe the project is wholesome or morally right or because they earn a tax deduction is immaterial. Similarly, it does not matter whether a politician supports a public health policy change because it will improve the health of the public or because it will win votes. What matters is that we have been effective in building relationships to mobilize support for a healthy community agenda. It is important to remember that what is "right" in community life is seldom black or white. Practically all people live in a world of shifting priorities and contradictions and claim a morality that they cannot possibly practice to its fullest. Most people, for example, endorse freedom of the press and the protection of individual privacy. If a highly regarded person is the subject of an unflattering front-page story, community residents may find themselves supporting the right to privacy. On the other hand, the same residents may invoke freedom of the press to publicly discredit a less highly regarded individual.

Advocates of the consensus model cite its unifying capacity, bringing various groups together to work for a common purpose, overcoming resistance to change, and developing a sense of pride in being part of something that is bigger than one's self or even one's family. Advocates of the conflict model contend that change achieved through consensus is often trivial and will have little impact on the social and economic dislocations that are at the root of poor health and health disparities. According to the conflict model, the reason people do not want to change is not because humans have an inherent resistance to doing so but because they have a vested interest in the status quo. Whether change is described as disorganizing or reorganizing depends on where one stands in the shifting control of resources. Consensus and conflict strategies each have a place in empowering groups to action, but when and how they are used should be grounded in the cultural information derived from the community assessment.

According to Gilles Bibeau (1997), the lack of success in health promotion and prevention in North America and throughout the world can be attributed to the failure to acknowledge the complexities of community culture and the reflexive endorsement of action strategies that make assumptions about cultural homogeneity in communities.

THE ROLE OF THE NURSE IN COMMUNITY ACTION

In clinical practice, nurses understand the significance of establishing relationships with their patients to increase the effectiveness of their interventions. But organizing whole communities for civic action offers a different set of challenges that reflect the complexity and diversity of community clients. Nurses are accustomed, for example, to establishing a sense of confidence and trust with patients and their families as they become active and essential participants in their care plans. In community health, it is equally imperative to establish a strong and trusting relationship with clients and to engage them in community action. But because communities are composed of competing populations, groups, and institutions, establishing a trusting relationship with one segment of the community could generate concern in another segment. Even the appearance of an exclusive affiliation with one community group could compromise one's effectiveness in working with the community as a whole. A community/public health nurse who routinely attends a Methodist church, for example, needs to demonstrate his or her respect for other religions in the town or neighborhood by meeting with their leaders and denominations.

Community practitioners become, in effect, ex-officio members of the community, but they are not just *any* members of the community. They occupy a special role, relative to other residents, that carries privileges and obligations. On the one hand, they have more personal freedom than other members of the community and typically are judged by a different set of standards. Nurses are permitted—even expected—to develop relationships with all members of the community, including vulnerable or "hidden" populations, such as the homeless, and to visit areas of the community that would be considered off-limits to some residents. They also are privileged to ask highly personal questions, explore the more intimate details of people's lives, and provide hands-on personal care. On the other hand, the nurse's position and special role within the community carries certain constraints and responsibilities. Because nurses are reservoirs of knowledge about the personal aspects of residents' lives, confidentiality of individual residents and of the community must be maintained. For example, it is a breach of confidentiality for the nurse to participate in the casual gossip and speculation afforded to most members of the community without seriously undermining the nurse's credibility and the community's trust.

Building community relations becomes even more complicated when community/public health nurses reside in the community where they work. As residents, nurses are complex stakeholders, ordinarily occupying several positions or roles that could result in conflicting allegiances. At the same time, being a resident can augment effectiveness. If community/public health nurses have children attending local schools, for example, they will have a personal as well as a professional interest in street safety and school health. If the owner of the local industry is a relative or a friend, the nurse may be well positioned to negotiate for occupational safety improvements. For community/public health nurses who reside in the communities where they work, community members are not just the target population; they are their children's teachers, their spouse's employer, their rabbi, or their mechanic. For the residents, the community/public health nurse is not just a nurse but also a neighbor, a customer, or a fellow club member. It is not impossible for nurses to balance and negotiate community relationships; it simply requires thoughtful consideration of their relationships with the individuals and groups that make up the population of the community.

Regardless of whether they are residents, the ultimate goal of community/public health practice is to build community capacity. In some respects, building community capacity is not unlike helping individuals and families acquire the skills to successfully manage the problems, losses, crises, and adjustments that are bound to occur over a lifetime. Unlike patients and families, however, communities are matrices where complex and often competing institutions and populations intersect. Community/public health nurses must work thoughtfully and skillfully with the full range of community leaders and institutions found in almost all communities.

CREATING A COMMUNITY ACTION PLAN FOR A HEALTHY COMMUNITY AGENDA

Chapter 7, "Laying the Foundation for a Healthy Community Agenda," took us from the overarching goal and vision of a prepared, sustainable community through the development of a culturally informed strategic plan for implementing public health objectives. In this chapter, we apply the findings of our community-culture inquiry and health assessment in the planning and implementation of a culturally informed community action plan. A *community action plan* (also called a *plan of work* or an *operational plan*) identifies the specific activities and events needed to achieve the overarching goals and objectives of the healthy community agenda. The community action plan translates program objectives into a community-specific plan of work in a detailed description of the what, who, when, and where of the initiative.

The Mobilize, Assess, Plan, Implement, Track (MAP-IT) framework for community action presented in *Healthy People 2020* is a useful guide for moving through the process of leading change. MAP-IT alone, however, will not provide the specific strategies required to build community capacity and mobilize civic action within the cultural context of a particular community. We may understand the meaning and importance of *mobilize*, for example, but how do we mobilize in Eau Claire, Wisconsin, as opposed to New Orleans, Louisiana, or Willits, California, or Shelburne Falls, Massachusetts, or Chicago's north side? To make MAP-IT come alive with the cultural realities of our specific community, the complexities and nuances of local life must be translated into each category of the framework.

Designing a culturally informed community action plan requires an analysis of the problem in relation to the context of community life:

- What is the nature and extent of the problem?

- How does the target population fit into community life?

- What is the community cultural capital that can be applied to this public health problem?

■ At what points do the special needs of the target population intersect with community institutions and populations?

■ What are the local barriers that will need to be addressed?

To illustrate, let's explore the process of developing a culturally informed community action plan using one of the new topic areas in *Healthy People 2020*: older adults.

As baby boomers (adults born between 1946 and 1964) age, they remain one of the fastest-growing age groups in the nation. Because of the advances in medical science, people in this age group are living longer, but they also are more likely to be living with at least one chronic illness. It is predicted that by 2030, more than 37 million baby boomers (60%) will be managing more than one chronic illness. Even though most older adults want to stay in their homes, chronic illness and injury (such as falls) may limit their capacity to remain independent. Prevention and health-promotion programs designed to prevent declines from illness and falls are supported by federal government agencies and are included in the Patient Protection and Affordable Care Act. Fewer than 20% of older adults, however, engage in physical activity (*Healthy People 2020*). Moreover, if they *do* acquire illnesses and disabilities, they may have insufficient support (coordination of care, public transportation, neighborhood safety, home reconfiguration, reliable caregivers, specially educated health professionals, and family and social networks) to continue living independently.

Even though states that invest in such services show lower rates of growth in long-term-care expenditures, the potentially soaring healthcare costs associated with expensive hospitalizations, long-term care, and rehabilitative services place an enormous burden on the healthcare system and provide a disincentive to allocate additional resources. Not surprisingly, the overarching goal for older adults in *Healthy People 2020*—to "improve the health, function, and quality of life of older adults"—involves 12 objectives in the areas of prevention and long-term services and supports:

■ Increase the proportion of older adults who use the "Welcome to Medicare" benefit.

- Increase the proportion of older adults who are up-to-date on a core set of clinical preventative services.

- (Developmental) Increase the proportion of older adults with one or more chronic health conditions who report confidence in managing their conditions.

- Increase the proportion of older adults who receive diabetes self-management benefits.

- Reduce the proportion of older adults who have moderate to severe functional limitations.

- Increase the proportion of older adults with reduced physical or cognitive function who engage in light, moderate, or vigorous leisure-time physical activities.

- Increase the proportion of the healthcare workforce with geriatric certification.

- (Developmental) Reduce the proportion of non-institutionalized older adults with disabilities who have an unmet need for long-term services and supports.

- (Developmental) Reduce the proportion of unpaid caregivers of older adults who report an unmet need for caregiver-support services.

- Reduce the rate of pressure-ulcer-related hospitalizations among older adults.

- Reduce the rate of emergency department visits due to falls among older adults.

- Increase the number of states and tribes (including the District of Columbia) that collect and make publicly available information on the characteristics of victims, perpetrators, and cases of elder abuse, neglect, and exploitation.

The health and quality of life of older adults is a nationwide issue, but its expression and extent will vary locally. Although programs offered by federal agencies provide many resources to address the concern, the most effective health promotion, prevention, and management solutions will be accomplished in the cultural context of communities where older adults live. A culturally informed community action plan that will accomplish the objectives and overarching goals outlined in

Healthy People 2020 begins with comparing and contextualizing the community's older adult population according to the three dimensions of community life:

- The physical environment of time and space

- The characteristics of the population

- The social relationships and interactions within the population and between the population and the environment

There are a number of ways to define the population in question, depending on the community as well as the problem. In the following example, the older adult population is divided into two subpopulations: people ages 65 to 79 and people ages 80 and older. Typically, concerns about living at home alone and the need for effective support services begin to intensify around age 80.

By plotting the two groups of older adults within the matrix of community culture, we secure a deeper understanding of the strength and the vulnerability of these two older adult populations and how they relate to the larger community. We then can see how our target population of interest intersects with the wider community. We discover the cultural capital—the people, institutions, services, and environmental features—that can be mobilized to create the most cost-effective, culturally informed community action plan.

- **The environment (place):** Where and when can we find our two groups of older adults in the community? Are they more likely to reside in specific neighborhoods or apartment complexes, or are they distributed evenly throughout the community? Where and when do they congregate (restaurants, faith-based institutions, Rotary or Lions Club meetings, recreational activities)? How do they use their time on a daily, weekly, and seasonal basis? For example, do they visit family every weekend? Do they leave (or return) for the winter months?

Suggested Activity

Analyze the identified community health issue or concern in relation to its cultural context.

Building Capacity for Healthy Aging: Culture Context Analysis

Objective: Increase the Percentage of Older Adults Who Reside Independently in Their Homes	Adults Ages 65–79	Adults Ages 80 and Older
Physical Environment: Space and Time		
Where do they live (which neighborhoods)?		
Where do they spend their day? Week? Year?		
Where and when do they go on a daily and weekly basis?		
Where and when do they get together?		
The Population		
What are the number and percentage of older adults in the community?		
What are the demographics?		
Age		
Sex		
Religion		
Ethnicity		
Class		
Residence		
Housing		
Length of time in the community		

Objective: Increase the Percentage of Older Adults Who Reside Independently in Their Homes	Adults Ages 65–79	Adults Ages 80 and Older
The Social System		
What is their relationship to community institutions?		
Religion		
Economy/workforce/job		
Recreation/sports		
Healthcare		
Education		
Domestic/family life		
Communication/ transportation		
Where do they fit into a horizontal stratification of the community?		
Where do they fit into a community vertical segmentation?		

- **The population (people):** How many persons in the community are in one of these two age groups? What is the percentage of older adults in the community? In what kind of housing do older adults live—in their own homes, with younger family members, in retirement communities, in assisted-living centers, in skilled-nursing facilities? How many live alone? How physically close are their families? What are the socio-demographic characteristics of this population (e.g., sex, ethnicity, class, religion, income, education, housing, and length of time in the community)?

- **The social organization:** Where do older adults fit into the socioeconomic stratification of the community? For example, are they equally distributed among the classes or do they, as a group, tend to represent the more powerful or least powerful strata of the community's class structure? Do they occupy a special segment of the community (e.g., long-time residents or newcomer retirees, a distinct ethnic category, a seasonal population)? In what ways do older adults participate in community life? What are the community services they use (e.g., grocery stores, hairdressers, public transportation, drugstores, dry cleaners, lawn services, legal services)? What are the forms of recreation in which they engage (e.g., television, bridge games, casinos, bingo, movies, operas and symphonies, the library, and recreational and fitness classes)?

From this cultural information about the role and status of our population of interest, we can begin to understand and address how they promote their own health and maintain their preferred lifestyles, such as living in their homes as long as possible. Who are the people who have a vested interest in their welfare (e.g., family members, religious leaders, neighbors, people who deliver the mail, friends, health insurers, hairdressers, grocers, lawn service, a local car service)? Is the restaurant where they gather a natural location in which to provide health education and group support? Will grocery stores provide shopping and transportation services? Each community will be very different in terms of the stakeholders involved and the kind of action required. Addressing the issue of residential living for older persons in a community where older adults are in daily physical contact with family members is very different from one in which their families live thousands of miles away. There will be different sets of stakeholders, different interventions, and different timeframes, reflecting the cultural distinctions of each community.

Today, intranet and visual computer technology makes it possible to connect older adults not only with their children and grandchildren but also with the services they need. As experts in the management of elder care, nurses can collaborate with experts in computer technology to build communication systems that permit even the frailest older adults to remain at home and in contact with the world.

No matter which organizational strategy or combination of strategies is used in public health, it must be grounded in the identification and application of community cultural capital (i.e., the values, beliefs, events, organizations, physical structures, and citizens required to build public health capacity). By articulating community health goals with the community's culture and sharing the responsibility for community health with designated community members, we can accomplish an effective and sustainable healthy community agenda. This is true whether the specific issue is senior living, child obesity, domestic violence, toxic waste, or summer-recreation safety.

When community action plans are culturally informed, the resulting changes are necessarily more sustainable and permanent, because they are embedded in the lifeways, values, and norms of the community. Plans consistent with the community's culture inspire the commitment and willingness of people and institutions to engage in policies and community action that perpetuate local values. External funding may be needed to initiate an action, but culturally informed plans are grounded in the cost-efficient strategy of deploying existing cultural capital for sustainable change. Effective and successful community action over time builds a community's capacity for health and well-being, thereby expanding useful cultural capital. When change occurs without cultural guidance, community-action efforts are at risk of not becoming fully incorporated into the culture of the community and may jeopardize the community's confidence in the public health practitioner.

THE MAP-IT FRAMEWORK: MOBILIZE, ASSESS, PLAN, IMPLEMENT, AND TRACK

Now you are ready to walk through a culturally informed version of the MAP-IT framework for community action.

MOBILIZE

Mobilizing for public health action is about identifying and building relationships with community stakeholders. Each objective in a healthy community agenda gives rise to two kinds of stakeholders, or target populations, needed to engage and accomplish the action plan. Those who are directly affected by the action plan constitute the *primary target*—the category of individuals or groups for whom the program is intended (e.g., senior citizens, migrant workers, or automobile drivers). The *secondary target* consists of those people and organizations that may not be affected by the program directly but are instrumental in facilitating (or impeding) its success. Legislators, for example, are an important secondary target group in sponsoring regulations that will provide safe housing for older adults. Factory owners may be a critical secondary target group for supporting elder day care programs for their employees who are caregivers of their elder parents. Children and schools could be secondary targets in a program to help children dissuade their grandparents from smoking. Secondary targets include community decision-makers whose endorsement is needed to accomplish the proposed plan as well as those who have a vested interest in the project.

The forum for mobilizing stakeholders for civic action is called a coalition. Unlike constituencies, which provide ongoing support and representation for nurses, a *coalition* is a group of individuals and organizations that has been convened for the express purpose of accomplishing a specific goal. The identification and selection of a coalition is drawn from our ethnographic analysis of the problem or issue in the context of the specific culture. Time, for example, is a critical consideration in identifying which legislator to include in the coalition. The choice of legislator will depend not only on voting histories and campaign promises but also on his or her term of office and proximity to the next election. A popular owner of a restaurant in which older adults gather routinely; the president of the Rotary Club, who may himself or herself be over age 65; a contractor who can retrofit homes with safety bars and ramps; and a computer programmer/educator who could help older adults access the Internet and communicate routinely with friends, families, and health providers are all potential coalition members.

Each coalition is composed of a different set of individuals, some of whom may be opponents on some issues but have come together for a cause they now have in common. For example, a Catholic priest and a state-government representative may work very well together in advancing the health and well-being of older citizens but be in completely different camps when it comes to contraception and sex education in schools. Coalitions are important not only for mobilizing community members around a particular initiative but also for establishing relationships where none existed previously and for engaging all citizens as stakeholders in building capacity. When individuals and groups that ordinarily are on opposite sides of the table have the opportunity to collaborate on a common cause, they also have the opportunity to develop personal relationships that may soften their disagreement on other issues.

Healthy People 2020 identifies four questions to ask and answer:

- What is the vision and mission of the coalition?

- Why do I want to bring people together?

- Who should be represented?

- Who are the potential partners (organizations and businesses) in my community?

Suggested Activity

Applying information from the analysis of the community culture inquiry, list six individuals and/or groups whom you could potentially invite to serve on a coalition to address your identified community health issue/problem. Identify the value each member brings as well as the potential difficulty each member may pose.

Coalition Membership	Position in Community and His/Her Value to the Initiative	Potential Barriers or Problems His/Her Presence May Create

ASSESS

One of the first responsibilities of the coalition members is to acquire an understanding of the problem, issue, or concern as it is expressed in the community, its determinants, and the resources available to address it. The focus should be on (a) who is affected and how, (b) what resources we have, and (c) what resources we need. For example:

- How large are the 65–79 and 80 and older populations now?

- What will they be in 5, 10, and 20 years?

- What are the percentages of these populations in relation to the population of the whole community?

- How do they compare to national, state, and local statistics? (This may be an indicator of the availability of national, state, and local resources.)

- How many and what percentage of older adults live at home or reside in assisted-living or long-term-care facilities?

- What are the number, purpose, and percentage of hospital admissions and emergency department visits?

- How many older adults admitted to the hospital end up never again living independently in their homes?

- How many older adults are at risk of having to leave their homes?

- What type and amount of resources are required to increase the number of older adults who reside in their own homes?

  - Physical reconfiguration of homes for easier access

  - Emergency-call capability

  - Computer and intranet communication devices

  - Reliable transportation

  - Personal shoppers

  - Visiting services

  - Assistance with paying bills and home management

■ What resources currently exist in the community to address the issue?

■ What programs/interventions have been used in other communities to address the same issue?

■ Review the best practices and evidence-based programs found in the literature for applicability. Are they consistent with the culture of this community and able to be translated into its values and lifeways?

■ What factors need to be identified or addressed to support sustainability?

The purposes of the assessment are as follows:

■ To identify the severity and extent of the issue or problem and its impact on local life

■ To identify the resources—or cultural capital—available to address the concern

■ To discern the applicability of tested programs in similar communities that have produced desired results

The assessment is necessary for prioritizing the action plan and revealing existing local resources that can be mobilized and directed to address the safety and independence of older citizens. Many resources may already exist within a community, but without a culture inquiry, they may not be immediately obvious. Here are a few examples:

■ In a hilly New England town, the community/public health nurse invited a local ski resort to donate its used ski poles so older adults could use them get outside during the winter.

■ In a southern community, high school seniors prepared a laminated list of important phone numbers in large print for older adults living at home and then helped them input the numbers into their phones' contact lists for direct dialing.

■ With the assistance of a local farmer who donated space in his barn, a community/public health nurse in a Midwest agricultural community created a storage area for used hospital beds, commodes, crutches, canes, and other medical equipment that could be distributed to community residents who needed them.

■ Nursing students assigned to manage the care of adults over age 80 who were living at home were able to reduce depression rates simply by calling three times a week to ask questions about their mobility, medication, and social activity.

Using the local cultural capital of a ski resort, a high school senior civics class, a retired farmer with a large barn, and a college nursing course in gerontology, these communities were able to offer sustainable, no-cost or low-cost contributions to the health and independence of older adults.

PLAN

Public health action would be simple if you could count on everyone in the community to see the importance and logic of supporting a particular initiative. In reality, however, practically all public health initiatives will be received with varying degrees of enthusiasm—from full support, to indifference, to frank opposition. The sequential steps of an action plan will identify the relationships and actions required for community support. Sometimes, opposition is the product of a simple lack of understanding of the project's mission and can be corrected easily with action steps focused on communication and education. Other times, opposition comes from competition for limited resources, in which case the action-step response may be a trade-off—for example, "I will support your school's lunch program if you support my program to offer vision screening for older adults." Reduced transit fares for people age 65 and older may require data about the costs to taxpayers when older adults are not able to live in their own homes.

Healthy People 2020 offers useful questions to ask when writing action steps, including the following:

■ What will happen?

■ Who will do what?

- When will it happen?

- What are the other resources required?

- What are the barriers and sources of resistance, and how will they be overcome?

- Who are the collaborators?

Suggested Activity

Using information from the community culture inquiry, write action steps using the *Healthy People 2020* guidelines to address the identified problem/issue. What factors need to be identified and addressed that demonstrate the reduced cost and sustainability of community action? Formulate a plan for demonstrating the sustainability of community action.

One of the most important responsibilities of a coalition is the formulation of the action plan to generate and debate ideas not only on steps and priorities but also on the suitability of best practices and interventions that have been used in other communities. Ample time, open discussion, and opportunities for changing the plan, if necessary, must be provided. Action plans must be fluid and flexible to accommodate changes in the problem and in the community and subject to revision as circumstances change. Every member of the coalition should have a copy of the most up-to-date version and be prepared to revisit it on a regular basis. The plan also must be unambiguous and measurable so that it is well understood and easily communicated and so that progress can be monitored routinely and revised, if necessary. The action steps should be the logical outcome of and reflect the overarching goal, vision, mission, objectives, and strategies of the plan.

Community Health Issue

Long-Term Goal

Short-Term Outcomes

**Potential Actions/
Intervention(s)**

Action Step	Person(s) Responsible	Date to Be Completed	Resources Required	Plan for Barriers and Resistance	Collaborators

IMPLEMENT

Successful implementation of a community action plan begins with acknowledging that some members of the community will support it, others will oppose it, and still others will not really care either way. Neglecting to identify those who are against or indifferent jeopardizes the initiative—particularly if the opposition is organizing for counteraction. It is important to know not only their reasons for resisting but also their influence within the community. Supporters and opponents are embedded in the social and economic structures that make up the local culture. By understanding these components of the culture, it is possible to construct trade-offs, compromises, or even win-wins that will satisfy everyone. A creative long-term-care facility, for example, could develop products and services that permit individuals to stay in their own homes as long as possible, while simultaneously cultivating the loyalty of individuals and families so that if and when they do need full-time skilled-nursing care, it will be in the facility of choice.

Organization for action requires equal attention to those who are "neutral" to the initiative. These are the groups and individuals that have—or believe they have—nothing to gain or lose in the proposed plan and are, therefore, indifferent. They should not be ignored: first, because support derived from the neutral group may be essential for the project's approval; and second, because irresolute individuals and groups could easily be persuaded to join the opposition. By including neutral but powerful individuals and organizations in the coalition, neutrality or apathy may be transformed into commitment. Again, allies, opponents, and neutrals do not remain the same but shift in relation to the specific initiative. Just because the bus-transit system supports a program for accommodating passengers with disabilities does not mean it will support a reduction in fares for older adults. The strategy in all community health planning is to articulate and balance competing segments of the community to accomplish a healthy community agenda. Compromise and trade-offs are at the heart of community/public health politics.

Most important, do not be persuaded by the inherent goodness of the initiative. It is unlikely that a particular behavior or institution could continue to flourish if someone did not stand to gain from it. It is better to anticipate opposition to even the most modest and seemingly rational change and to prepare for it accordingly. Finally, it is not unusual for opposition to come from health-professional organizations that have a vested interest in maintaining existing services. School nurses, for example, have reported encountering opposition from pediatricians to school-based health programs that offer free sports physicals.

TRACK

According to *Healthy People 2020*, as the action plan is implemented, it is important to review whether you are following the plan and what you can do better. Having an evaluation plan to track implementation of the healthy community agenda is essential to assess progress, analyze trends over time, and evaluate program objectives and progress toward the long-term goals. In clinical practice, measuring such criteria as body temperature, redness, or swelling tells us whether the treatment for infection has been effective. This also is true of community/public health practice. Once the action plan has been identified and endorsed, the coalition must decide on measurable targets, including how progress will be measured, a timeline for measurement, and the procedures that will be employed. Compared with clinical practice, however, these outcomes include community (e.g., capacity, infrastructure, cultural capital), system (e.g., development sustainability, flexibility, cost), and, when appropriate, individual health measures. Additionally, the length of time ordinarily required to see results from community interventions is much longer than the length of time for outcomes measurement in clinical practice.

Healthy People 2020 identifies questions that should be answered in a plan for regular evaluations to track implementation of the action plan:

- Are we evaluating our work?

- Did we follow the plan?

- What did we change?

- Did we reach our goal?

Additionally, if appropriate, it is important to ask what efforts are in place to promote sustainability and what risks need to be identified to ensure that community-action efforts are maintained.

Suggested Activity

Based on your community culture and health assessments, identify short-term outcomes and long-term goals to meet the healthy community agenda.

Action Plan Activities	Short-Term Outcomes to Meet Activity Objectives	Short-Term Outcome Measures	Dates to Be Completed	Long-Term Goal	Long-Term Goal Measures	Date to Be Completed

Process evaluation occurs throughout the implementation of the healthy community agenda and provides the opportunity to change the direction of initiatives and interventions if they are not going as expected, effects are untoward, resources change, expectations are not being met, or other strategies are deemed more appropriate to the community. *Outcome evaluation*, on the other hand, is centered on the achievement of the healthy community agenda goals and outcomes.

Although evaluation is often portrayed as occurring after the plan is in place and underway, in actuality, process- and outcome-evaluation criteria are identified and incorporated into the plan early and throughout the process.

Finally, the objectives and strategies of a healthy community agenda should offer the most cost-effective, and thus sustainable, solution to the problem. Cost-effectiveness is not synonymous with least expensive. Rather, it gives consideration to the relationship between cost and quality. For one intervention to be considered more cost-effective than another, it must provide equal outcomes at a lower cost or better outcomes at the same cost. Cost must be measured not only in terms of dollars and cents but also in the hidden expenditures of productivity, time, and psychological tolls that are more difficult to monetize. The initial expense for a project may be high, but sustainability may require less investment. On the other hand, a plan with lower startup costs could ultimately prove to be a more expensive, less sustainable alternative in the long run. It could be argued, for example, that a preliminary analysis of the community's culture is too time-consuming. Yet a plan that is consistent with the cultural expectations and conditions of the community can avoid time-consuming and expensive mistakes. All cost calculations must include the costs incurred if such a program were *not* implemented.

Northville and Southfield: Examples of Culturally Informed Community Action

A comparison of two communities, fictitiously called Northville and Southfield, located in the same rural county, reveals the ways in which the positions and roles of the target groups in their communities influence the configuration of an action plan that is part of a healthy community agenda, including the coalition, the assessment data, the short- and long-range activities, the implementation strategies, and the metric to be achieved.

Nurses from the county decided to seek fiscal support from its 20 towns to extend health-promotion, preventive, and health-maintenance services to the growing population of older adults. Each of the towns already provided a range of well-child services, administered by community/public health nurses. The services included postnatal visits to high-risk families, parenting classes, child-development programs, and nutrition programs as well as immunizations, physical exams, and auditory and vision screenings. These programs were administered in collaboration with the schools and supported with funds derived partly from the state and partly from the collection of town tax revenues. The proposed plan would expand public health services to older adults and add health education, recreational programs, and community safety to the annual flu-prevention programs.

Southfield is a rural farming community with a population of about 2,100 people, of which almost 300 are age 65 or older. Northville, a neighboring community, has a population of about 2,600, of which approximately 250 are age 65 or older. In spite of the demographic similarities between the towns and their geographic proximity, the proposal for a commitment to elder services was accepted readily by elected officials in Southfield but rejected in Northville.

An examination of the role and status of the older adult population (the primary target) in each community provides some clues to explain the difference in commitment to the program by each community. Southfield is a farming community in which older adults continue to work in some capacity on family-operated farms, assuming household and child-care responsibilities. Although they may be less active than their children and/or grandchildren in farm operations, they typically are the owners of the farms that succeeding generations will inherit. For the most part, the social life of Southfield is intergenerational and organized around the network of extended families that compose the population of the town. In addition to their central economic roles as owners of the farms, older adults continue to take active roles as leaders in town government, church functions, and community social activities, such as the annual fair or the annual pancake breakfast sponsored by the volunteer firefighters.

Northville resembles Southfield in physical appearance and would be classified as rural by most standards. Only a small segment of the Northville population still engages in farming, however. Most of the land is rented to farmers in surrounding communities, such as Southfield. Much of the population is employed at the large, prestigious Valley Preparatory School tucked into the hills surrounding the center of town. Because residence in Northville entitles local children to tuition benefits as day students at Valley School, many young families have moved to Northville but commute daily to work in the county seat, located 15 miles away. A few of the older adults in this community are senior members of farm families, as in Southfield, but most are retired members of the faculty and staff from the preparatory school. Unlike the older adults in Southfield, most Northville older adults live far from their sons and daughters, who typically live in other parts of the country. The social and recreational activities in Northville are much more age-segregated, so the various generations mix only infrequently. Although the retirees and the younger men engage in golf as a pastime, the older adults use a local nine-hole course, while the younger men travel to a more sophisticated golf club in the county seat that puts them in contact with their daily business associates.

In comparison with the Southfield older adults, those in Northville are not well integrated with the other generations. They play almost no role in town government, which generally is controlled by the younger generation, and have little economic authority in the community. Older adults simply are not a high priority in Northville. There is even occasional resentment expressed regarding older adult residents who continue to occupy large homes in a community where spacious houses are much in demand by young families with children. Essentially, Northville older adults have less authority and fewer advocates than their Southfield counterparts.

This example demonstrates that it is not just the size and nature of the target group that matter but its role and status in relation to the rest of the community—particularly the power structure. In Southfield, where older adults were comparatively powerful, town officials readily accepted and implemented the proposal. In Northville, on the other hand, the retired members of the community had no clearly visible support base, so the first step was to identify those groups and individuals who would constitute a coalition.

An analysis of the position of elder community members in relation to the cultural context of Northville revealed various points at which older adults did, in fact, intersect with other age groups. First, although they were not great in number, grandparents and great-grandparents played significant roles in a few extended farm families. Second, the Congregational Church, in which some retired faculty members from Valley School served as Sunday School teachers, was one of the few community domains in which intergenerational activities and relationships had developed and flourished—particularly among the women. Third, as the leader of a major "industry" in Northville, the headmaster of Valley School was considered to be one of the more influential members of the community.

From this analysis, a Northville coalition was formed that included the following people:

- The minister of the Congregational Church

- A well-liked mother whose child attended Sunday School at the church and whose husband happened to be an elected town official

- A respected farmer whose extended family, including his father, lived on the family farm

- An articulate retired Valley School faculty member

Together, they visited the headmaster of Valley School to ask for his support in convincing town-council members to provide revenue for the project. His own political leverage stemmed from the school's role as a major employer in the community and from its generous tuition benefits to town children. In the meantime, the wife of the town official convinced her husband to reverse his original opinion on the project, and the much-beloved and highly influential minister asked his parishioners for their endorsement. By developing a strategy grounded in knowledge of community culture, this strategically selected coalition was able to overcome the original opposition and secure the resources needed to acquire the commitment of town revenues for promoting the health of older adults.

FORMULATING A CULTURALLY EFFECTIVE COMMUNITY CASE STATEMENT

In clinical practice, nurses present their care plans in a manner that will ensure their patients' understanding of the importance of the treatment and their engagement. This requires individualizing the plan so it is consistent with the lifestyle and values of the specific patient and his or her family. Similarly, to convince a community to embrace system-level action, we must construct a message that is framed within the cultural experience of the community. The goal is to create awareness in the community to generate public action. Whether we are trying to improve the living conditions of seasonal workers, manage solid waste, or limit smoking in public places, community consciousness raising will be necessary. Climate change, school violence, child obesity, HIV/AIDS, disaster preparedness, and violence against women have captured the attention of the public, creating a demand for their resolution. Not surprisingly, simply creating a healthy future for the community may not be a sufficiently powerful motivator for public action without specific action objectives (e.g., better schools for children, improved public transportation, beautification of the downtown area, safer neighborhoods) that will resonate with the community members. The argument that automobile emissions are contributing to the gradual reduction of the ozone layer, for example, simply may not be as compelling to individuals and families as the prospect of losing jobs within the next 6 months because of new regulations governing the disposal of industrial wastes.

Given the diversity of the community and the presence of proponents, opponents, and neutrals in almost all capacity-building agendas, effective community appeal will likely have to contain more than one message. Some sectors of the community, for example, will respond very well to the argument that regulating the disposal of industrial wastes will result in a healthier environment for future generations. Others will see such an effort as endangering their economic livelihoods by regulating the industries in which they work. In a diverse community, the message and the action plan must be segmented to address the various goals and values present in the community we are attempting to persuade.

In addition to a culturally appropriate and segmented message, the culturally effective community case statement must include all the critical information related to the issue in culturally informed communication strategies so that everyone who is promoting the community action is well prepared to defend it—especially members of the coalition. In explaining their support of controversial legislation, politicians, for example, must have compelling justification regarding the costs as well as the benefits to their constituents to ensure the sustainability of the initiative.

The community case statement for sustainability consists of the following:

- The overarching goal, which the action plan supports

- A statement of the problem (what is the issue/concern?)

- The magnitude of the problem (the number and characteristics of the individuals and families in the community who are or will be affected—directly and indirectly)

- The cost of the issue/problem to the community (what is the impact, and at what cost?)

- Cost of the proposed action

- The projected outcomes

- The cost to the community of *not* taking this action

The community case statement is generated by the coalition and then designed and used to inform all relevant segments of the community so that everyone involved will be working toward the same goal with the same information, even if it might be for different reasons.

The goal of the case statement is to convince and persuade; therefore, all information must be accurate, reliable, and understandable to all segments of the community. Statistics and statements of fact must be current and compiled from credible sources, checked, and rechecked. Even the most minor math error detracts from the credibility of the document and its authors. Because those who are not in favor of the proposed change may examine the statement carefully in an attempt to discredit the message, the facts must be accurate and the argument logical to defend the statement and counter opposition.

Finding the proper balance between statistical data and qualitative descriptions will depend on the characteristics of the audience. Because we live in a society that has confidence in science and numbers, statistical evidence is useful but should be selected carefully to make the point. Less scientific, but sometimes more convincing, are human-interest stories that have an emotional appeal. A description of one or two actual cases will be highly persuasive, especially when combined with a statistical analysis of hundreds of families. Thus, although it is necessary to have an objective, rational argument about why a specific plan would improve the health of the community, an emotional appeal can be extraordinarily effective, even with the most conservative audience. For example, although the millions of tax dollars spent on drug-abuse interdiction and treatment each year are compelling, they are somehow less real than the case of a family who lost its home and savings because of drug abuse by one of its members. The plight of real people is something with which almost everyone can identify.

In conclusion, the overarching goal of public health practice is a healthy community—with the capacity to mobilize cultural capital to protect the growth, sustainability, and equity of community life. Although much of public health practice is focused on the action plan, the strategy for achieving our overarching goal is not just implementing a collection of unrelated community initiatives but rather an integrated, comprehensive, culturally informed healthy community agenda.

REFERENCES

Acevedo-Garcia, D., Lochner, K. A., Osypuk, T. L., & Subramanian, S. V. (2003). Future directions in residential segregation and health research: A multilevel approach. *American Journal of Public Health, 93*(2), 215–220.

Alinsky, S. (1971). *Rules for radicals*. New York, NY: Vintage Books, Random House.

American Lung Association. (2010). *State of the air 2010: Key findings*. Retrieved from http://stateoftheair.org/

American Nurses Association. (2007). *Public health nursing: Scope and standards of practice*. Silver Spring, MD: Author.

American Nurses Association. (2015). *What is nursing?* Retrieved from http://nursingworld.org/EspeciallyForYou/What-is-Nursing

Andrews, M., & Boyle, J. (2008). *Transcultural concepts in nursing care*. Philadelphia, PA: Lippincott Williams and Wilkins.

Arensberg, C. (1954). The community study method. *American Journal of Sociology, 60*(2), 109–124.

Arensberg, C. (1955). American communities. *American Anthropologist, 57*(6), 1143–1162. Doi: 10.1525/aa.1955.57.6.02a00060

Arensberg, C. (1961). The community as object and sample. *American Anthropologist, 63*(2), 241–264. Doi: 10.1525/aa.1961.63.2.02a00010

Arensberg, C., & Kimball, S. (1965). *Culture and community*. New York, NY: Harcourt, Brace, and World.

Armelagos, G. J., Brown, P. J., & Turner, B. (2005). Evolutionary, historical and political economic perspectives on health and disease. *Social Science and Medicine, 61*(4), 755–765. Doi: 10.1016/j.socscimed.2004.08.066

Bender, A., Clune, L., & Guruge, S. (2009). Considering place in community health nursing. *Canadian Journal of Nursing Research, 41*(1), 128–143.

Benkert, R., Tanner, C., Guthrie, B., Oakley, D., & Pohl, J. M. (2005). Cultural competence of nurse practitioner students: A consortium's experience. *Journal of Nursing Education, 44*(5), 225–233.

Berkman, L. F., & Syme, S. L. (1979). Social networks, host resistance, and mortality: A nine-year follow-up study of Alameda County residents. *American Journal of Epidemiology, 109*(2), 186–204.

Bernard, H. R. (2011). *Research methods in anthropology: Qualitative and quantitative approaches* (5th ed.). Lanham, MD: AltaMira Press.

Betancourt, J. R., Green, A. R., Carrillo, J. E., & Ananeh-Firempong, O., 2nd. (2003). Defining cultural competence: A practical framework for addressing racial/ethnic disparities in health and health care. *Public Health Reports, 118*(4), 293–302.

Bibeau, G. (1997). At work in the fields of public health: The abuse of rationality. *Anthropology Quarterly, 11*(2), 246–252. Doi: 10.1525/maq.1997.11.2.246

Bloom, B., Cohen, R., & Freeman, G. (2009). *Summary health statistics for U.S. children: National health interview survey, 2008.* National Center for Health Statistics, Vital Health Statistics. Series 10, No. 244: 1–81.

Bonnie, R. J., & Wallace, R. B. (Eds.). (2003). *Elder mistreatment: Abuse, neglect, and exploitation in an aging America: Panel to review risk and prevalence of elder abuse and neglect.* Washington, DC: National Academies Press.

Boonn, A. (2015). *State cigarette excise tax rates and rankings.* Retrieved from https://www.tobaccofreekids.org/research/factsheets/pdf/0097.pdf

Buhler-Wilkerson, K. (1993). Bringing care to the people: Lillian Wald's legacy to public health nursing. *American Journal of Public Health, 83*(12), 1778–1786.

Burgard, S. A., Brand, J. E., & House, J. S. (2007). Toward a better estimation of the effect of job loss on health. *Journal of Health and Social Behavior, 48*(4), 369–384. Doi: 10.1177/002214650704800403

Butterfield, P. (1990). Thinking upstream: Nurturing a conceptual understanding of the societal context of health behavior. *Advances in Nursing Science, 12*(2), 1–8.

Butterfield, P. (2002). Upstream reflections on environmental health: An abbreviated history and framework for action. *Advances in Nursing Science, 25*(1), 32–49.

Campinha-Bacote, J., & Munoz, C. (2001). A guiding framework for delivering culturally competent services in case management. *The Case Manager, 12*(2), 48–52. Doi: 10.1067/mcm.2001.114902

Carlson, E., & Chamberlain, R. (2004). The black-white perception gap and health disparities research. *Public Health Nursing, 21*(4), 372–379. Doi: 10.1111/j.0737-1209.2004.21411.x

Carolan, M., Andrews, G. J., & Hodnett, E. (2006). Writing place: A comparison of nursing research and health geography. *Nursing Inquiry, 13*(3), 203–219. Doi: 10.1111/j.1440-1800.2006.00322.x

Case, A., & Deaton, A. (2015). *Rising morbidity and mortality in midlife among white non-Hispanic Americans in the 21st century.* Proceedings of the National Academy of Sciences, 1–6. Retrieved from www.pnas.org/cgi/doi/10.1073/pnas.1518393112

Centers for Disease Control and Prevention, Core Public Health Functions Steering Committee. (2010a). *National public health performance standards program: Orientation to the essential public health services.* Retrieved from http://www.cdc.gov/nphpsp/essentialServices.html

Centers for Disease Control and Prevention. (2010b). *Racial and ethnic minority populations.* Retrieved from http://www.cdc.gov/minorityhealth/index.html

Centers for Disease Control and Prevention, National Center for Injury Prevention and Control. (2011). *Web-based injury statistics query and reporting system (WISQARS).* Retrieved from http://www.cdc.gov/injury/wisqars

Centers for Disease Control and Prevention. (2011). *Chronic disease prevention and health promotion.* Retrieved from http://www.cdc.gov/chronicdisease/index.htm

Centers for Disease Control and Prevention. (2012). *Asthma.* Retrieved from http://www.cdc.gov/nchs/fastats/asthma.htm

Centers for Disease Control and Prevention. (2013). *The state of aging and health in America 2013.* Retrieved from http://www.cdc.gov/features/agingandhealth/state_of_aging_and_health_in_america_2013.pdf

Centers for Disease Control and Prevention. (2015). *Climate and health.* Retrieved from http://www.cdc.gov/climateandhealth

Centers for Disease Control and Prevention. (2016). *Morbidity and mortality weekly report (MMWR).* Retrieved from http://www.cdc.gov/mmwr/index.html

Centers for Disease Control and Prevention. (n.d.). *Community health in action.* Retrieved from http://www.cdc.gov/nccdphp/dch

Chafey, K. (1996). "Caring" is not enough: Ethical paradigms for community-based care. *Nursing and Health Care Perspectives on Community, 17*(1), 10–15.

City-Data.com. (n.d.). *Races in Cloudcroft, New Mexico (NM) detailed stats.* Retrieved from http://www.city-data.com/races/races-Cloudcroft-New-Mexico.html

Civic Impulse. (2016). H.R. 3590–111th Congress: *Patient protection and affordable care act.* Retrieved from https://www.govtrack.us/congress/bills/111/hr3590

Clancy, K. J., Berger, P. D., & Magliozzi, T. L. (2003). The ecological fallacy: Some fundamental research misconceptions corrected. *Journal of Advertising Research, 43*(4), 370–380.

Clark, M. (2007). *Community health nursing: Advocacy for population health,* 5th ed. Upper Saddle River, NJ: Prentice Hall.

Corin, E. (1994). The social and cultural matrix of health and disease. In R. G. Evans, M. L. Barer, & T. R. Marmor (Eds.), *Why are some people healthy and others not? The determinants of health of populations,* 93–132. Hawthorne, NY: Aldinede Gruyter.

Cummins, S., Curtis, S., Diez-Roux, A. V., & Macintyre, M. (2007). Understanding and representing "place" in health research: A relational approach. *Social Science and Medicine, 65*(9), 1825–1838. Doi: 10.1016/j.socscimed.2007.05.036

Cummins, S., Stafford, M., Macintyre, S., Marmot, M., & Ellaway, A. (2005). Neighborhood environment and its association with self-rated health: Evidence from Scotland and England. *Journal of Epidemiology and Community Health, 59*(3), 207–213. Doi: 10.1136/jech.2003.016147

Cuzick, J. (2003). Epidemiology of breast cancer—selected highlights. *Breast, 12*(6), 405–411. Doi: 10.1016/S0960-9776(03)00144-9

Davis, R. (2000). Holographic community: Reconceptualizing the meaning of community in an era of health care reform. *Nursing Outlook, 48*(6), 295–301. Doi: 10.1067/mno.2000.107152

Dreher, M. (1982a). The conflict of conservatism in public health nursing education. *Nursing Outlook, 30*(9), 504–509.

Dreher, M. (1982b). *Working men and ganja.* Philadelphia, PA: ISHI Publications.

Dreher, M. (1984). District nursing: The cost benefits of a community-based practice. *American Journal of Public Health, 74*(10), 1107–1111.

Dreher, M. (1996). Nursing: A cultural phenomenon. *Reflections on Nursing Leadership, 22*(4), 4.

Dreher, M., & Hudgins, R. (2010). Maternal conjugal multiplicity and child development in rural Jamaica. *Family Relations, 59*(5), 495–505. Doi: 10.1111/j.1741-3729.2010.00617.x

Dreher, M., & MacNaughton, N. (2002). Cultural competence in nursing: Foundation or fallacy? *Nursing Outlook, 50*(5), 181–186.

Dressler, W. W. (1982). *Hypertension and culture change: Acculturation and disease in the West Indies.* South Salem, NY: Redgrave.

Dressler, W. W. (1985). The social and cultural context of coping: Action, gender, and symptoms in a southern black community. *Social Science and Medicine, 21*(5), 499–506. Doi: 10.1016/0277-9536(85)90033-4

Dressler, W. W. (2004). Culture and the risk of disease. *British Medical Bulletin, 69*(1), 21–31. Doi: 10.1093/bmb/ldh020

Drevdahl, D. (1995). Coming to voice: The power of emancipatory community interventions. *Advances in Nursing Science, 18*(2), 13–24.

Drevdahl, D. (1999). Meanings of community in a community health center. *Public Health Nursing, 16*(6), 417–425. Doi: 10.1046/j.1525-1446.1999.00417.x

Drevdahl, D. J. (2002). Home and border: The contradictions of community. *Advances in Nursing Science, 24*(3), 8–20.

Drevdahl, D., Philips, D., & Taylor, J. (2006). Uncontested categories: The use of race and ethnicity variables in nursing research. *Nursing Inquiry, 13*(1), 53–63. Doi: 10.1111/j.1440-1800.2006.00305.x

Dubos, R. (1965). *Man adapting.* New Haven, CT: Yale University Press.

DuRant, R. H., Cadenhead, C., Pendergrast, R. A., Slavens, G., & Linder, C. W. (1994). Factors associated with the use of violence among urban black adolescents. *American Journal of Public Health, 84*(4), 612–617.

Eberhardt, M., & Pamuk, E. (2004). The importance of place of residence: Examining health in rural and non-rural areas. *American Journal of Public Health, 94*(10), 1682–1686.

Edelson, M. (2008). Culturally attuned messages delivered by peers may be the best way to stop HIV from surging among at-risk, hidden populations. *Johns Hopkins Public Health Magazine.* Retrieved from http://magazine.Jhsph.edu/2008/Spring/culture/living

Epps, F. R., Skemp, L., & Specht, J. (2015). Using culturally informed strategies to enhance recruitment of African Americans in dementia research: A nurse researcher's experience. *Journal of Research Practice, 11*(1), Article M2. Retrieved from http://jrp.icaap.org/index.php/jrp/article/view/512/416

Everly, G. S., Jr., & Flynn, B. W. (2006). Principles and practical procedures for acute psychological first aid training for personnel without mental health experience. *International Journal of Emergency Mental Health, 8*(2), 93–100.

Fahrenwald, N., Boysen, R., Fischer, C., & Maurer, R. (2001). Developing cultural competence in the baccalaureate nursing student: A population-based project with the Hutterites. *Journal of Transcultural Nursing, 12*(1), 48–55. Doi: 10.1177/104365960101200107

Fahrenwald, N., Taylor, J., Kneipp, S., & Canales, M. (2007). Academic freedom and academic duty to teach social justice: A perspective and pedagogy for public health nursing faculty. *Public Health Nursing, 24*(2), 190–197. Doi: 10.1111/j.1525-1446.2007.00624.x

Feld, M. (2008). *Lillian Wald: A biography.* Chapel Hill, NC: University of North Carolina Press.

Fisher, T. L., Burnet, D., Huang, E., Chin, M., & Cagney, K. (2007). Cultural leverage: Interventions using culture to narrow racial disparities in health care. *Medical Care Research Review, 64*(5 Suppl), 243S–282S. Doi: 10.1177/1077558707305414

Freeman, R. (1963). *Public health nursing practice* (3rd ed.). Philadelphia, PA: Saunders.

Friedman, T. (2008). *Hot, flat and crowded.* New York, NY: Farrar, Straus, and Giroux.

Gehlbach, S. (2005). *American plagues: Lessons from our battles with disease.* New York, NY: McGraw-Hill Professional.

Glied, S., & Ma, S. (2015). How will the Affordable Care Act affect the use of healthcare services? *Issue Brief* (*The Commonwealth Fund*), Pub. 1804. Vol. 4. Retrieved from http://www.commonwealthfund.org/~/media/files/publications/issue-brief/2015/feb/1804_glied_how_will_aca_affect_use_hlt_care_svcs_ib_v2.pdf

Grunberg, L., Moore, S., Greenberg, E. S., & Sikora, P. (2008). The changing workplace and its effects: A longitudinal examination of employee responses at a large company. *Journal of Applied Behavioral Science, 44*(2), 215–236. Doi: 10.1177/0021886307312771

Hammett, T. M., Harmon, M. P., & Rhodes, W. (2002). The burden of infectious disease among inmates of and releases from U.S. correctional facilities, 1997. *American Journal of Public Health, 92*(11), 1789–1794.

Hebel, J. R., & McCarter, R. J. (2006). *A study guide to epidemiology and biostatistics* (6th ed.). Sudbury, MA: Jones and Bartlett Learning.

Helman, C. (2007). *Culture, health, and illness*. London, England: Hodder Arnold.

Henry Street Settlement. (n.d.). *Lillian Wald*. Retrieved from http://www.henrystreet.org/about/history/lillian-wald.html

Heymann, J., Hertzman, C., Barer, M., & Evans, R. (2006). *Healthier societies: From analysis to action*. Oxford, England: Oxford University Press.

Hopkins, N., & Mehanna, S. R. (2000). Social action against everyday pollution in Egypt. *Human Organization, 59*(2), 245–254.

Hopkins, N., & Mehanna, S. R. (2003). Living with pollution in Egypt. *The Environmentalist, 23*(1), 17–28.

Institute of Medicine. (2008). *Retooling for an aging America: Building the health care workforce*. Washington, DC: National Academies Press.

Institute of Medicine. (2010). *The future of nursing: Leading change, advancing health*. Washington, DC: National Academies Press.

Kaiser Family Foundation. (2006). *Fact sheet: Young African American men in the United States*. Retrieved from http://www.kff.org/minorityhealth/upload/7541.pdf

Keene, D., Padilla, M., & Geronimus, A. (2010). Leaving Chicago for Iowa's "fields of opportunity": Community dispossession, rootlessness, and the quest for somewhere to "be OK." *Human Organization, 69*(3), 275–284.

Kerker, B., Bainbridge, J., Kennedy, J., Bennani, Y., Agerton, T., Marder, D., ... Thorpe, L. (2011). A population-based assessment of the health of homeless families in New York City, 2001–2003. *American Journal of Public Health, 101*(3), 545–553. Doi: 10.2105/AJPH.2010.193102

Kleinman, A. (1980). *Patients and healers in the context of culture*. Berkeley, CA: University of California Press.

Koplan, J. P., Bond, T. C., Merson, M. H., Reddy, K. S., Rodriguez, M. H., Sewankambo, N. K., ... Wasserheit, J. N. (2009). Towards a common definition of global health. *Lancet, 373*(9679), 1993–1995. Doi: 10.1016/S0140-6736(09)60332-9

Krause, N. (2002). Church-based social support and health in old age: Exploring variations by race. *Journals of Gerontology. Series B, Psychological Sciences and Social Sciences, 57*(6), S332–347. Doi: 10.1093/geronb/57.6.S332

Kreuter, M., & McClure, S. (2004). The role of culture in health communication. *Annual Review of Public Health, 25*, 439–455. Doi: 10.1146/annurev.publhealth.25.101802.123000

KU Work Group for Community Health and Development. (2015). *The community tool box*. University of Kansas. Retrieved from http://ctb.ku.edu

Kung, H. C., Hoyert, D. L., Xu, J., & Murphy, S. L. (2008). Deaths: Final data for 2005. *National Vital Statistics Reports, 56*(10). Retrieved from http://www.cdc.gov/nchs/data/nvsr/nvsr56/nvsr56_10.pdf

Leininger, M. (1988). Leininger's theory of nursing: Cultural care diversity and universality. *Nursing Science Quarterly, 1*(4), 152–160. Doi: 10.1177/089431848800100408

Leininger, M. (1997). Transcultural nursing research to transform nursing education and practice: 40 years. *Journal of Nursing Scholarship, 29*(4), 341–348. Doi: 10.1111/j.1547-5069.1997.tb01053.x

Levine, A. (1982). *Love canal: Science, politics, and people*. Lexington, MA: Lexington Books.

Levy, B., & Sidel, V. (2006). *Social injustice and public health*. New York, NY: Oxford University Press.

Marmot, M. (2005a). The social environment and health. *Clinical Medicine, 5*(3), 244–248.

Marmot, M. (2005b). Social determinants of health inequalities. *Lancet, 365*(9464), 1099–1104. Doi: 10.1016/S0140-6736(05)71146-6

McElroy, A., & Townsend, P. (2004). *Medical anthropology in ecological perspective*. New York, NY: Westview Press.

McKay, M. L., & Hewlett, P. O. (2009). Grassroots coalition building: Lessons from the field. *Journal of Professional Nursing, 25*(6), 352–357. Doi: 10.1016/j.profnurs.2009.10.010

McMichael, A. J. (2001). *Frontiers, environments, and disease: Past patterns, uncertain futures.* Cambridge, England: Cambridge University Press.

Milio, N. (1970). *9226 Kercheval Street: The storefront that did not burn.* Ann Arbor, MI: University of Michigan Press.

Milio, N. (1975). *The care of health in communities.* New York, NY: MacMillan.

Minkler, M. (2005). *Community organizing and community building for health.* Newark, NJ: Rutgers University Press.

National Alliance on Mental Illness. (2013). *Mental illness facts and numbers.* Retrieved from http://www2.nami.org/factsheets/mentalillness_factsheet.pdf

National Center for Health Statistics. (2012). *Health, United States 2011: With special feature on socioeconomic status and health.* Hyattsville, MD: Centers for Disease Control and Prevention.

National Heart, Lung, and Blood Institute and Boston University. (2011). *Framingham heart study.* Retrieved from http://www.framinghamheartstudy.org

National Institutes of Health. (n.d.). *Toxnet toxicology data network: Welcome to Toxnet.* Retrieved from http://toxnet.nlm.nih.gov

Newton, L., & Smith, D. (2004). *Wake-up calls: Classic cases in business ethics.* Mason, OH: Thomson/South-Western.

Office of National Drug Control Policy. (2000, March). *Drug-related crime.* Retrieved from http://docplayer.net/5561718-Ondcp-drug-policy-information-clearinghouse-fact-sheet-john-p-walters-director-www-whitehousedrugpolicy-gov-1-800-666-3332-drug-related-crime.html

Office of National Drug Control Policy. (2006). *Drug policy information clearinghouse fact sheet.* Retrieved from http://www.whitehousedrugpolicy.gov/publications/factsht/crime/index.html

Ogden, C., & Carroll, M. (2010). *Prevalence of obesity among children and adolescents: United States, trends 1963–1965 through 2007–2008.* Centers for Disease Control and Prevention. Retrieved from http://www.cdc.gov/nchs/data/hestat/obesity_child_07_08/obesity_child_07_08.htm

Ogden, C., Carroll, M., Kit, B., & Flegal, K. (2014). Prevalence of childhood and adult obesity in the United States, 2011–2012. *Journal of the American Medical Association, 311*(8), 806–814. Doi: 10.1001/jama.2014.732

Omeri, A., & Malcolm, P. (2004). Cultural diversity: A challenge for community nurses. *Contemporary Nurse, 17*(3), 183–191.

Paul, B. (Ed.). (1955). *Health, culture, community: Case studies of public reactions to health programs.* New York, NY: Russell Sage Foundation.

Peterson, J., Atwood, J., & Yates, B. (2002). Key elements for church-based health promotion programs: Outcome-based literature review. *Public Health Nursing, 19*(6), 401–411. Doi: 10.1046/j.1525-1446.2002.19602.x

Phillips, D., & Drevdahl, D. (2003). "Race" and the difficulties of language. *Advances in Nursing Science, 26*(1), 17–29.

Pobutsky, A. M., Baker, K. K., & Reyes-Salvail, F. (2015). Investigating measures of social context on 2 population-based health surveys, Hawaii, 2010–2012. *Preventing Chronic Disease, 12,* E221. Doi: 10.5888/pcd12.150319

Population Reference Bureau. (2015). *Population of youth ages 10–24.* Retrieved from http://www.prb.org/DataFinder/Topic/Rankings.aspx?ind=19

Public Health Foundation (PHF). (2011). *Quad Council public health nursing competencies.* Retrieved from http://www.phf.org/resourcestools/Pages/Public_Health_Nursing_Competencies.aspx

Public Health Foundation. (2014). Core competencies for public health. Retrieved from http://www.phf.org/resourcestools/Pages/Core_Public_Health_Competencies.aspx

Putic, G. (2014). African media try to educate public about ebola. *Voice of America*. Retrieved from http://www.voanews.com/content/African-media-tries-to-educate-public-about-ebola/2422696.html

Quad Council of Public Health Nursing Organizations. (2004). Public health nursing competencies. *Public Health Nursing, 21*(5), 443–452. Doi: 10.1111/j.0737-1209.2004.021508.x

Racher, F., & Annis, R. (2007). Respecting culture and honoring diversity in community practice. *Research and Theory in Nursing Practice, 2*(14), 255–270.

Reagan, P. B., & Salsberry, P. J. (2005). Race and ethnic differences in determinants of preterm birth in the USA: Broadening the social context. *Social Science and Medicine, 60*(10), 2217–2228. Doi: 10.1016/j.socscimed.2004.10.010

Roberts, E. (1997). Neighborhood social environments and the distribution of low birthweight in Chicago. *American Journal of Public Health, 87*(4), 597–603.

Rodwin, V., & Neuberg, L. (2005). Infant mortality and income in 4 world cities: New York, London, Paris, and Tokyo. *American Journal of Public Health, 95*(1), 86–90. Doi: 10.2105/AJPH.2004.040287

Rosen, G. (1954). The community and the health officer: A working team. *American Journal of Public Health Nations Health, 44*(1), 14–17.

Rothman, J. (Ed.). (2008). *Strategies of community intervention.* Peosta, IA: Eddie Bowers Pub.

Rowland, D. (2012). *Population aging: The transformation of societies.* In J. L. Powell & S. Chen (Series Eds.), *International Perspectives on Aging.* London, England: Springer Press.

Sikora, P., Moore, S., Greenberg, E., & Grunberg, L. (2008). Downsizing and alcohol use: A cross-lagged longitudinal examination of the spillover hypothesis. *Work and Stress, 22*(1), 51–68. Doi: 10.1080/02678370801999651

Simmons, A., Reynolds, R., & Swinburn, B. (2011). Defining community-capacity building: Is it possible? *Preventive Medicine, 52*(3–4), 193–199. Doi: 10.1016/j.ypmed.2011.02.003

Skemp Kelley, L. (2005a). Growing old in St. Lucia: Expectations and elder care networks in a St. Lucian village. *Journal of Cross-Cultural Gerontology, 20*, 67–78.

Skemp Kelley, L. (2005b). Gendered elder care exchanges in a Caribbean village. *Western Journal of Nursing Research, 27*(1), 73–92.

Skemp Kelley, L. (2005c). Minor children and adult care exchanges with community dwelling frail elders in a St. Lucian village. *Journal of Gerontology: Social Sciences, 60B*(2), S62–S73.

Skemp, L., Maas, M., & Umbarger-Mackey, M. (2014). Doing it my way. *The Gerontologist.* Doi: 10.1093/geront/gnt052

Stafford, M., & Marmot, M. (2003). Neighbourhood deprivation and health: Does it affect us all equally? *International Journal of Epidemiology, 32*(3), 357–366. Doi: 10.1093/ije/dyg084

Steckler, A. B., & Herzog, W. T. (1979). How to keep your mandated citizen board out of your hair and off your back: A guide for executive directors. *American Journal of Community Health, 69*(8), 809–812.

Strawbridge, W., Cohen, R., Shema, S., & Kaplan, G. (1997). Frequent attendance at religious services and mortality over 28 years. *American Journal of Public Health, 87*(6), 957–961.

Szwarcwald, C. L., da Mota, J. C., Damacena, G. M., & Pereira, T. G. (2011). Health inequalities in Rio de Janeiro, Brazil: Lower healthy life expectancy in socioeconomically disadvantaged areas. *American Journal of Public Health, 101*(3), 517–523. Doi: 10.2105/AJPH.2010.195453

Tarlier, D., Browne, A. J., & Johnson, J. (2007). The influence of geographical and social distance on nursing practice and continuity of care in a remote First Nations community. *Canadian Journal of Nursing Research, 39*(3), 126–148.

Tripp-Reimer, T. (1999). Cultural interventions for ethnic groups of color. In A. S. Hinshaw, S. Feetham, & J. Shaver (Eds.), *Handbook of clinical nursing research,* 107–123. Thousand Oaks, CA: Sage.

Tripp-Reimer, T., Choi, E., Skemp Kelley, L., & Enslein, J. (2001). Cultural barriers to care: Inverting the problem. *Diabetes Spectrum, 14*(1), 13–22.

United Nations Department of Economic and Social Affairs. (2010). *Water scarcity. International decade for action: Water for life, 2005–2015.* Retrieved from http://www.un.org/waterforlifedecade/scarcity.html

U.S. Census Bureau. (2008a). *2008 American community survey.* Retrieved from http://www2.census.gov/programs-surveys/acs/methodology/questionnaires/2008/quest08.pdf

U.S. Census Bureau. (2008b). *Population estimates: National characteristics: National sex, age, race, and Hispanic origin.* Retrieved from http://www.census.gov/popest/

U.S. Census Bureau. (2016). *American factfinder: Community facts.* Retrieved from http://factfinder.census.gov/faces/nav/jsf/pages/index.xhtml

U.S. Department of Health and Human Services (USDHHS). (2000). *Healthy People 2010.* Washington, DC: U.S. Government Printing Office.

U.S. Department of Health and Human Services. (2001). *Cultural competence works: Using cultural competence to improve the quality of health care for diverse populations and add value to managed care arrangements.* Merrifield, VA: LTG Associates, Inc., HRSA Information Center.

U.S. Department of Health and Human Services (USDHHS). (2010). *Healthy People 2020—Improving the health of Americans.* Retrieved from http://www.healthypeople.gov

U.S. Department of Health and Human Services. Office of Minority Health. (2010). *The national plan for action draft.* National Partnership for Action to End Health Disparities. Retrieved from http://www.minorityhealth.hhs.gov/npa/templates/browse.aspx?&lvl=2&lvlid=34

U.S. Environmental Protection Agency. (n.d.). *Toxics release inventory (TRI) program.* Retrieved from http://www.epa.gov/tri

University of Kansas. (2015). *Enhancing cultural competence.* Retrieved from http://ctb.ku.edu/en/enhancing-cultural-competence

Wald, L. (1915). *The house on Henry Street.* New York, NY: Henry Holt and Company.

Wald, L. (1934). *Windows on Henry Street.* Boston, MA: Little, Brown and Company.

Webb, B., Simpson, S., & Hairston, L. (2011). From politics to parity: Using a health disparities index to guide legislative efforts for health equity. *American Journal of Public Health, 101*(3), 554–559. Doi: 10.2105/AJPH.2009.171157

Wellin, E. (1955). *Water boiling in a Peruvian town. Health, culture, and community.* New York, NY: Russell Sage Foundation.

Whitaker, E. D. (2003). The idea of health: History, medical pluralism, and the management of the body in Emilia-Romagna, Italy. *Medical Anthropology Quarterly, 17*(3), 348–375. Doi: 10.1525/maq.2003.17.3.348

White, K. L. (1973). Life and death and medicine. *Scientific American, 229*(3), 23–33.

Whitehouse.gov. (2012). *The Obama administration and community health centers.* Retrieved from https://www.whitehouse.gov/sites/default/files/05-01-12_community_health_center_report.pdf

Williamson, M., & Harrison, L. (2010). Providing culturally appropriate care: A literature review. *International Journal of Nursing Studies, 47*(6), 761–769. Doi: 10.1016/j.ijnurstu.2009.12.012

Wolf, E. (1994). Perilous ideas: Race, culture, people. *Current Anthropology, 35*(1), 1–12.

Woodruff, T. J., Zota, A. R., & Schwartz, J. M. (2011). Environmental chemicals in pregnant women in the United States: NHANES 2003–2004. *Environmental Health Perspectives, 119*(6), 878–885. Doi: 10.1289/ehp.1002727

World Health Organization. (2007). *Global age-friendly cities: A guide.* Retrieved from http://www.who.int/ageing/publications/Global_age_friendly_cities_Guide_English.pdf

World Health Organization. (2011). *Ageing.* Retrieved from http://www.who.int/topics/ageing/en

World Health Organization. (2015). *World report on ageing and health.* Retrieved from http://www.who.int/ageing/publications/world-report-2015/en/

Worthman, C. M., & Kohrt, B. (2005). Receding horizons of health: Biocultural approaches to public health paradoxes. *Social Science and Medicine, 61*(4), 861–878. Doi: 10.1016/j.socscimed.2004.08.052

Young Laing, B. (2009). A critique of Rothman's and other standard community organizing models: Toward developing a culturally proficient community organizing framework. *Community Development, 40*(1), 17–20.

INDEX

A

H

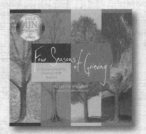
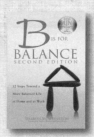
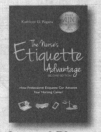
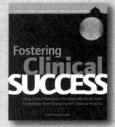
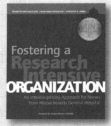
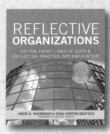
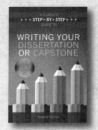

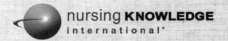

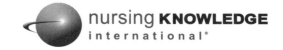

POPULATION-BASED PUBLIC HEALTH CLINICAL MANUAL
The Henry Street Model for Nurses
Second Edition

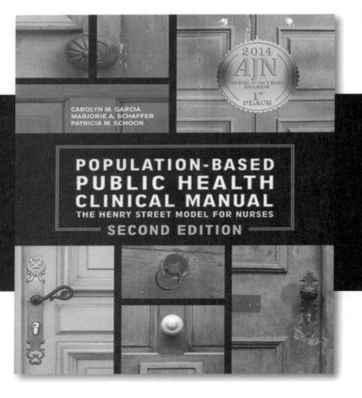

Carolyn M. Garcia
Marjorie A. Schaffer
Patricia M. Schoon

To order, visit **www.nursingknowledge.org/sttibooks**.
Discounts are available for institutional purchases. Call **888.NKI.4YOU** for details.

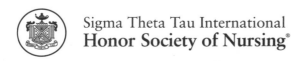

Sigma Theta Tau International
Honor Society of Nursing®

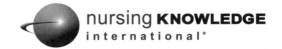

nursing **KNOWLEDGE**
international®